NATIONAL ACADEMIES

Sciences
Engineering
Medicine

NATIONAL
ACADEMIES
PRESS
Washington, DC

Dietary Patterns to Prevent and Manage Diet-Related Disease Across the Lifespan

Megan Snair, *Rapporteur*

Food Forum

Food and Nutrition Board

Health and Medicine Division

Proceedings of a Workshop

NATIONAL ACADEMIES PRESS 500 Fifth Street, NW Washington, DC 20001

This activity was supported by contracts between the National Academy of Sciences and National Institutes of Health (HHSN263201800029I /75N98023F00028); the U.S. Department of Agriculture (59-8040-3-001 and 123A9423P0005); and the U.S. Food and Drug Administration (75F40120C00192), with additional support from the American Heart Association; American Society for Nutrition; Cargill, Inc.; Center for Science in the Public Interest; The Coca-Cola Company; Conagra Brands; Danone North America; General Mills, Inc.; Institute of Food Technologists; Mars, Inc.; Mondelēz International; National Council on Aging; and Ocean Spray Cranberries, Inc. Any opinions, findings, conclusions, or recommendations expressed in this publication do not necessarily reflect the views of any organization or agency that provided support for the project.

International Standard Book Number-13: 978-0-309-71659-8
International Standard Book Number-10: 0-309-71659-4
Digital Object Identifier: https://doi.org/10.17226/27539

This publication is available from the National Academies Press, 500 Fifth Street, NW, Keck 360, Washington, DC 20001; (800) 624-6242 or (202) 334-3313; http://www.nap.edu.

Printed in the United States of America.

Suggested citation: National Academies of Sciences, Engineering, and Medicine. 2024. *Dietary patterns to prevent and manage diet-related disease across the lifespan: Proceedings of a workshop.* Washington, DC: The National Academies Press. https://doi.org/10.17226/27539.

The **National Academy of Sciences** was established in 1863 by an Act of Congress, signed by President Lincoln, as a private, nongovernmental institution to advise the nation on issues related to science and technology. Members are elected by their peers for outstanding contributions to research. Dr. Marcia McNutt is president.

The **National Academy of Engineering** was established in 1964 under the charter of the National Academy of Sciences to bring the practices of engineering to advising the nation. Members are elected by their peers for extraordinary contributions to engineering. Dr. John L. Anderson is president.

The **National Academy of Medicine** (formerly the Institute of Medicine) was established in 1970 under the charter of the National Academy of Sciences to advise the nation on medical and health issues. Members are elected by their peers for distinguished contributions to medicine and health. Dr. Victor J. Dzau is president.

The three Academies work together as the **National Academies of Sciences, Engineering, and Medicine** to provide independent, objective analysis and advice to the nation and conduct other activities to solve complex problems and inform public policy decisions. The National Academies also encourage education and research, recognize outstanding contributions to knowledge, and increase public understanding in matters of science, engineering, and medicine.

Learn more about the National Academies of Sciences, Engineering, and Medicine at **www.nationalacademies.org**.

Consensus Study Reports published by the National Academies of Sciences, Engineering, and Medicine document the evidence-based consensus on the study's statement of task by an authoring committee of experts. Reports typically include findings, conclusions, and recommendations based on information gathered by the committee and the committee's deliberations. Each report has been subjected to a rigorous and independent peer-review process and it represents the position of the National Academies on the statement of task.

Proceedings published by the National Academies of Sciences, Engineering, and Medicine chronicle the presentations and discussions at a workshop, symposium, or other event convened by the National Academies. The statements and opinions contained in proceedings are those of the participants and are not endorsed by other participants, the planning committee, or the National Academies.

Rapid Expert Consultations published by the National Academies of Sciences, Engineering, and Medicine are authored by subject-matter experts on narrowly focused topics that can be supported by a body of evidence. The discussions contained in rapid expert consultations are considered those of the authors and do not contain policy recommendations. Rapid expert consultations are reviewed by the institution before release.

For information about other products and activities of the National Academies, please visit www.nationalacademies.org/about/whatwedo.

PLANNING COMMITTEE FOR A WORKSHOP ON DIETARY PATTERNS TO PREVENT AND MANAGE DIET-RELATED DISEASE ACROSS THE LIFESPAN[1]

ROBIN A. McKINNON (*Chair*), Senior Advisor for Nutrition Policy, Center for Food Safety and Applied Nutrition, U.S. Food and Drug Administration

ALISON BROWN, Program Director, National Heart, Lung, and Blood Institute, National Institutes of Health

CINDY DAVIS, National Program Leader for Human Nutrition, Agricultural Research Service, U.S. Department of Agriculture

MARIO FERRUZZI, Professor and Section Chief, Arkansas Children's Nutrition Center, Department of Pediatrics, University of Arkansas for Medical Sciences, Director, USDA-ARS Arkansas Children's Nutrition Center

EMILY OKEN, Alice Hamilton Professor, Department of Population Medicine; Director, Division of Chronic Disease Research Across the Lifecourse, Harvard Medical School; Professor, Department of Nutrition, Harvard T.H. Chan School of Public Health; Vice Chair and Director of Faculty Development, Harvard Pilgrim Health Care Institute

REBECCA SEGUIN-FOWLER, Associate Director, Institute for Advancing Health through Agriculture; Chief Scientific Officer, Healthy Texas Institute, Texas A&M AgriLife; Professor of Nutrition, College of Agriculture and Life Sciences, Texas A&M University

JESSICA SMITH, Senior Principal Scientist, Nutrition, Scientific and Regulatory Affairs, Mars Wrigley North America

FANG FANG ZHANG, The Neely Family Professor and Associate Professor, Interim Chair, Division of Nutrition Epidemiology and Data Science, Friedman School of Nutrition Science and Policy, Tufts University

---

[1] The National Academies of Sciences, Engineering, and Medicine's planning committees are solely responsible for organizing the workshop, identifying topics, and choosing speakers. The responsibility for the published Proceedings of a Workshop rests with the workshop rapporteur and the institution.

FOOD FORUM (AS OF AUGUST 2023)[1]

ERIC A. DECKER (*Chair*), University of Massachusetts Amherst
RODOLPHE BARRANGOU, North Carolina State University, Raleigh
WENDY ATTAYA BOLAND, Kogod School of Business, American University, Washington, DC
CINDY DAVIS, Agricultural Research Service, U.S. Department of Agriculture, Beltsville, Maryland
DENISE R. EBLEN, Food Safety and Inspection Service, U.S. Department of Agriculture, Washington, DC
EMILY DIMIERO, Federal Government Relations, Cargill, Washington, DC
NAOMI K. FUKAGAWA, Agricultural Research Service, U.S. Department of Agriculture, Beltsville, Maryland
JAIME J. GAHCHE, Office of Dietary Supplements, National Institutes of Health, Bethesda, Maryland
CUTBERTO GARZA, Cornell University, Ithaca, New York
STEPHANIE K. GOODWIN, Danone North America, Washington, DC
M. R. C. GREENWOOD, University of California, Davis
MARTIN HAHN, Hogan Lovells, Washington, DC
BRYAN HITCHCOCK, Institute of Food Technologists, Chicago, Illinois
TERRY T-K HUANG, City University of New York School of Public Health and Health Policy, New York City
EVA HURT, The Coca-Cola Company, Atlanta, Georgia
RENÉE S. JOHNSON, Congressional Research Service, Library of Congress, Washington, DC
CHRISTINA KHOO, Ocean Spray Cranberries, Inc., Lakeville, Massachusetts
ALICE H. LICHTENSTEIN, Tufts University, Boston, Massachusetts
PETER LURIE, Center for Science in the Public Interest, Washington, DC
MEGAN NECHANICKY, General Mills, Inc., Golden Valley, Minnesota
RONI NEFF, Johns Hopkins University, Baltimore, Maryland
SAM R. NUGEN, Cornell University, Ithaca, New York
SARAH OHLHORST, American Society for Nutrition, Rockville, Maryland
HALEY F. OLIVER, Purdue University, West Lafayette, Indiana
DONALD A. PRATER, Center for Food Safety and Nutrition, U.S. Food and Drug Administration, College Park, Maryland

---

[1] The National Academies of Sciences, Engineering, and Medicine's forums and roundtables do not issue, review, or approve individual documents. The responsibility for the published Proceedings of a Workshop rests with the workshop rapporteur and the institution.

JILL REEDY, Division of Cancer Prevention, National Cancer Institute, National Institutes of Health, Bethesda, Maryland
KRISTIN REIMERS, Conagra Brands, Omaha, Nebraska
BRIAN RONHOLM, Consumer Reports, Washington, DC
SHARON A. ROSS, Division of Cancer Prevention, National Cancer Institute, National Institutes of Health, Bethesda, Maryland
SYLVIA B. ROWE, SR Strategy, LLC, Washington, DC
JENNIFER SALLIT, Mondelēz International, Orefield, Pennsylvania
JESSICA SMITH, Mars Wrigley North America, Hackettstown, New Jersey
PAMELA STARKE-REED, Agricultural Research Service, U.S. Department of Agriculture, Beltsville, Maryland
MARY T. STORY, Duke University, Durham, North Carolina
PATRICK J. STOVER, Texas A&M University, College Station
CHERYL TONER, American Heart Association, Washington, DC
DOROTHEA K. VAFIADIS, National Council on Aging, Arlington, Virginia

Health and Medicine Division Staff

HEATHER DEL VALLE COOK, Director, Food Forum
CYPRESS LYNX, Associate Program Officer
MEREDITH PARR, Research Assistant
ANN L. YAKTINE, Director, Food and Nutrition Board

Reviewers

This Proceedings of a Workshop was reviewed in draft form by individuals chosen for their diverse perspectives and technical expertise. The purpose of this independent review is to provide candid and critical comments that will assist the National Academies of Sciences, Engineering, and Medicine in making each published proceedings as sound as possible and to ensure that it meets the institutional standards for quality, objectivity, evidence, and responsiveness to the charge. The review comments and draft manuscript remain confidential to protect the integrity of the process.

We thank the following individuals for their review of this proceedings:

ALEXANDRA "LEXI" MacMILLAN URIBE, Texas A&M University
PAMELA STARKE-REED, U.S. Department of Agriculture
FANG FANG ZHANG, Tufts University

Although the reviewers listed above provided many constructive comments and suggestions, they were not asked to endorse the content of the proceedings, nor did they see the final draft before its release. The review of this proceedings was overseen by **ANNA MARIA SIEGA-RIZ,** University of Massachusetts Amherst. She was responsible for making certain that an independent examination of this proceedings was carried out in accordance with standards of the National Academies and that all review comments were carefully considered. Responsibility for the final content rests entirely with the rapporteur and the National Academies.

Contents

1

Introduction

The increasing rate of chronic disease in the United States has become a persistent, complex problem in the past few decades, one not easily solved. As researchers, health care providers, policy makers, community organizations, and various stakeholders seek to improve the health of individuals and communities, the role of diet in chronic disease has become an important area for exploration. Accordingly, on August 15–16, 2023, the Food Forum of the National Academies of Sciences, Engineering and Medicine held a workshop titled Dietary Patterns to Prevent and Manage Diet-Related Disease across the Lifespan.[1,2] In her introductory remarks, workshop planning committee chair Robin A. McKinnon, U.S. Food and Drug Administration, observed that research shows that current dietary patterns in the United States are not aligned with recommendations (see Figure 1-1). "As a population," she noted, "we underconsume vegetables, fruit, and whole grains but exceed recommended intakes for things such as added sugars and saturated fats, which collectively has implications for health and health care costs." She also highlighted the impact of this underlying

---

[1] The workshop agenda, presentations, and other materials are available at https://www.nationalacademies.org/event/40430_08-2023_dietary-patterns-to-prevent-and-manage-diet-related-disease-across-the-lifespan-a-workshop (accessed September 21, 2023).

[2] The planning committee's role was limited to planning the workshop, and the Proceedings of a Workshop was prepared by the workshop rapporteur as a factual summary of what occurred at the workshop. Statements, recommendations, and opinions expressed are those of individual presenters and participants and are not necessarily endorsed or verified by the National Academies of Sciences, Engineering, and Medicine, and they should not be construed as reflecting any group consensus.

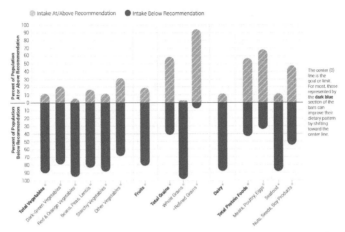

FIGURE 1-1 Dietary intake compared with recommendations: Percentage of individuals in the U.S. population aged 1 year and older who are below and at or above each dietary goal. SOURCES: Presented by Robin A. McKinnon on August 15, 2023. Reprinted with permission from the U.S. Department of Agriculture and the U.S. Department of Health and Human Services.

morbidity, which became apparent during the COVID-19 pandemic, when individuals with preexisting symptoms had a greater risk of severe disease and death. She also emphasized the complexity of understanding the many factors contributing to access to healthy food and informed food choices.

For the purposes of this workshop and in accordance with the Dietary Guidelines Advisory Committee (2020), McKinnon defined "dietary patterns" as the combination of an individual's complete dietary intake over time, as a description of a customary way of eating, or as a combination of foods recommended for consumption. She explained further that there are many diet-related diseases, but for this workshop speakers would focus on diseases linked to the highest rates of morbidity and mortality in the United States, including cardiovascular disease, diabetes, obesity, and certain cancers. Additionally, while physical activity is an important modifiable risk factor that influences diet-related disease outcomes, the workshop would be focused on dietary patterns and would not address physical activity. McKinnon also explained that while "food as medicine" initiatives would be included in the discussion, the workshop would not cover medically tailored meals, nor would it cover any topics under consideration by the 2025 Dietary Guidelines Advisory Committee. Finally, McKinnon highlighted the cross-cutting themes that would be highlighted throughout the workshop: equity, data quality and the current evidence base, policy challenges and opportunities, technology, and communications.

Discussions on day 1 of the workshop included dietary assessment; novel biomarkers for assessing dietary quality; and how diet influences the developmental origins of chronic disease, as well as the multitude of modifiable influences on dietary patterns and how they affect chronic disease risk and susceptibility (Chapter 2). Speakers also discussed the existing inequities in nutrition and food choice (Chapter 3) and the potential to influence these inequities through changes from industry and behavioral economics (Chapter 4). Day 2 of the workshop focused on perspectives on translating science into practice to improve adherence to dietary guidance, highlighting examples of organizations working to advance the health of communities through legal and policy opportunities for intervention (Chapter 5). The statement of task for the workshop is presented in Box 1-1. The workshop agenda, acronyms and abbreviations used in this publication, and biographical sketches of the workshop speakers and planning committee members can be found in Appendixes A, B, and C, respectively.

BOX 1-1
Statement of Task

A planning committee of the National Academies of Sciences, Engineering, and Medicine will organize a public workshop that will explore the state of the science around dietary patterns and diet-related chronic disease etiology, prevention, and management throughout the lifespan, including the developmental origins of disease. Workshop presenters, with multi-sector perspectives, will also discuss emerging research methodologies and technologies for assessing dietary patterns and connections to diet-related chronic disease at different life stages, including priorities for improving data gaps, and addressing barriers to innovation.

The planning committee will define the specific topics to be addressed, develop the workshop agenda, and select and invite speakers and discussants. A proceedings of a workshop in brief and full proceedings of the presentations and discussions at the workshop will be prepared by a designated rapporteur.

2

Setting the Stage on Dietary
Patterns and Chronic Disease

The speakers in the first session, moderated by Cindy Davis, U.S. Department of Agriculture, reviewed historical methods for assessing dietary patterns and discussed the potential for using more dynamic methods to better characterize a healthy dietary trajectory across the life course. Speakers also examined potential dietary biomarkers, reviewed the evidence connecting diet to chronic disease, and shared an evolutionary biology perspective on the developmental origins of health and disease.

DIETARY PATTERN ASSESSMENT ACROSS THE LIFE COURSE

Jill Reedy, National Institutes of Health, began by reviewing use of the evidence base generated from analyses of single nutrients to determine the relationship between diet and health outcomes. She characterized this as a reductionist approach, however, as nutrients and foods are seldom eaten in isolation, and there are many potential synergies among dietary components. Therefore, she suggested, an alternative, integrative approach would consider the effects of whole eating patterns. She recounted efforts over the past decade to synthesize evidence, define dietary patterns, advance assessment methods, and draft frameworks for studying the food supply at all levels. Specifically, she said, researchers have been considering how best to conceptualize diet as a multidimensional behavior and exposure.

According to Reedy, this shift began when the *2010 Dietary Guidelines for Americans* (DGA) report drew attention to dietary patterns; however, she said, the committee found it difficult to draw conclusions about the role of dietary patterns in health outcomes because of varying analytical approaches, which typically fall into three categories: data driven (such as factor analysis and cluster analysis), investigator driven (such as diet quality index scores), and hybrid (such as reduced-rank regression). In 2012, the International Conference on Diet and Activity Methods focused on how to advance the assessment of dietary patterns. Reedy pointed out that most research to this point had focused on the single dimension of what food is eaten. The draft framework developed by the conference encompassed multiple layers across the food supply, capturing not only what is eaten but also when, where, why, and how. Reedy explained that at this time, researchers became increasingly aware that individuals cannot be expected to make healthy choices if those options are not readily available.

Subsequently, Reedy continued, the Dietary Patterns Methods Project was established, with the goal of strengthening evidence and establishing a systematic method for analyzing dietary patterns ahead of the forthcoming revision of the DGA. Working with various large cohorts to achieve sufficient power, researchers found common underlying constructs across four selected indices: the Healthy Eating Index (HEI), the Alternative HEI, the Alternate Mediterranean Diet Score, and the Dietary Approaches to Stop Hypertension (DASH) score. Despite differences in methods, dietary components examined, and scoring approaches, Reedy said, the researchers found that higher diet quality was associated with lower mortality across three distinct cohorts and all four indices (Liese et al., 2015). This study therefore showed that there are multiple ways to eat a healthy diet and provided an opportunity to use dietary patterns to inform policy makers and guideline developers.

In 2015, Reedy reported, the Dietary Guidelines Advisory Committee used dietary patterns as the core of its conceptual model and framed its findings accordingly, while also noting that the components of an overall diet may have synergistic and cumulative effects on health and disease. According to Reedy, this shift in thinking was pivotal in influencing how the DGA would be framed going forward. The focus of subsequent committee deliberations began to shift from simply tracking what food components are being eaten to considering eating frequency and time-restricted eating. The recommendations of the most recent DGA are presented by life stage and include discussion of a healthy eating trajectory, she added. There is great interest in this idea of a healthy eating trajectory across the life course, she noted, and she displayed a figure showing dietary trajectories through different life-course stages (Figure 2-1), a perspective that helps identify target points for intervention and how they might be used in models with healthy outcomes. To this point, for example, the HEI originally covered only ages 2 years and older, but it now includes ages 12 to 23 months, providing new considerations for the early stage of healthy eating. The first 2 years of life is a period of rapid growth and development, Reedy observed,

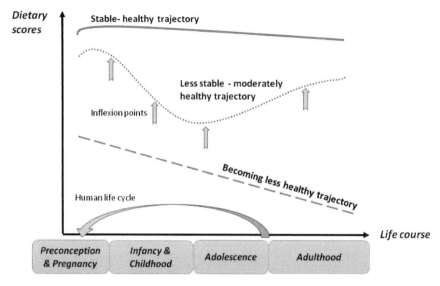

FIGURE 2-1 Dietary trajectories through different life stages.
SOURCES: Presented by Jill Reedy on August 15, 2023, from Chong, 2022. Reprinted with permission from Cambridge University Press.

so thinking about how to conceptualize and assess dietary intake in this stage is an important opportunity.

Reedy shared another way to visualize and assess dietary patterns by considering different components that underlie a total score and using that information in modeling. Figure 2-2, based on data from the National Health and Nutrition Examination Survey, 2011–2018, shows 13 components depicted on a spider web graph, plotted along its axis as a percentage of its maximum points, from 0 to 100 percent. She explained that a perfect score reflects optimal alignment with recommendations, with intake of components recommended for moderate consumption (saturated fats, added sugars, sodium, and refined grains) being low and intake of all other components being high. For toddlers aged 12 to 23 months, she elaborated, the score was higher for components such as total and whole fruits, dairy foods, and total protein foods, but lower for whole grains and total vegetables. The scores continued to decrease for each adolescent age group. For adults, the 19- to 59-year-old group had suboptimal scores, but a slight increase was observed for the age 60 and older group.

Lastly, Reedy presented a case study for the first 6 months of life, assessing the recommendation to feed infants exclusively human milk (or formula when human milk is unavailable) and exploring ways to answer questions of what, when, where, why, and who. Many surveys are not

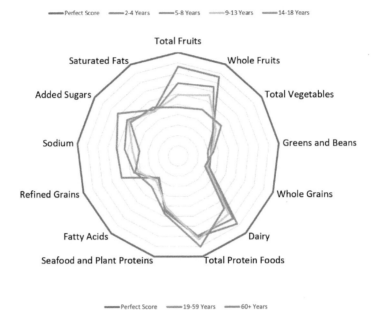

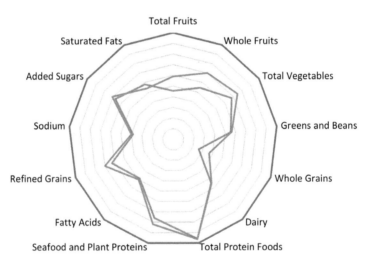

FIGURE 2-2 Healthy Eating Index-2020 radar plots across the lifespan, National Health and Nutrition Examination Survey, 2011–2018.
SOURCES: Presented by Jill Reedy on August 15, 2023, data from Herrick et al., 2023; Lerman et al., 2023; Pannucci et al., 2023; and Shams-White et al., 2023.

asking these questions, she said, even though they have the tools to do so. The questions are relevant in all life stages, she observed, but this context is even more important for children in the first 2 years of life. While much of the work in nutrition has focused historically on optimizing nutrients as the primary exposure, she stressed the potential of incorporating other data layers, such as temporal eating patterns; behavioral factors, which can be captured using innovative technology; and geospatial coding.

In summary, Reedy highlighted opportunities and challenges to consider when measuring and modeling the multiple dimensions of dietary patterns at different life stages. She gave the examples of using a shared conceptual framework across research questions, developing methods and models that fully capture total dietary patterns at different life stages, considering the timing and frequency of dietary patterns, and applying systems-oriented approaches that take into account measures of related exposures and their interactions within the context of dietary patterns.

BEYOND TRADITIONAL NUTRITION MARKERS FOR ASSESSING DIETARY QUALITY AND CHRONIC DISEASE RISK

The human diet is an extremely complex exposure, said Johanna Lampe, Fred Hutchinson Cancer Center, and when it comes to understanding the effects of diet on chronic disease, it is necessary to think about the totality of diet. The simpler dietary assessment instruments are, the more potential there is for bias and inaccuracies in measurement, she added, so more approaches are needed to help objectively capture dietary intake. Lampe pointed to dietary biomarkers as a way to provide a more objective evaluation of exposure to nutrients and dietary constituents, validate dietary assessments, calibrate dietary intake data, and establish biological links. Complementing the development of dietary biomarkers over the past decades, she observed, has been the development of -omics technologies, which allow analysis of up to thousands of compounds in a biologic sample, even making it possible to look at the impact of diet on the microbiome.

Lampe shared some examples of applications of dietary pattern biomarkers to illustrate approaches being used and opportunities for their expansion. She focused mainly on studies of standardized dietary patterns with the goal of evaluating the association between dietary patterns and biomarkers. First, she reviewed work from the American Cancer Society looking at a serum untargeted metabolomic profile in a cancer prevention cohort (McCullough et al., 2019). The researchers found varying metabolites, and the different diet pattern indices used also showed differences in the kinds of metabolites captured. For example, the HEI captured several phytochemicals (labeled as xenobiotics) found in various foods. However, Lampe explained, many metabolites have yet to be identified in these untargeted metabolomics platforms, so gaps in knowledge persist as to what compounds help define different diet scores. She added that, looking at predicting adherence to a healthy dietary pattern, these researchers found that just having data on more metabolites is not necessarily better for prediction; in some cases, data on just one or two metabolites can be as useful for predicting adherence as having data on all of them available.

The gut microbiome is also emerging as a way to monitor diet quality, Lampe continued, as there is an association between diet quality and fecal microbial diversity: greater diversity is typically a marker of a healthy microbiome and is often achieved through higher fruit and vegetable intake. Most analyses characterizing gut microbial activity are conducted using stool samples, she pointed out, characterizing this as a limitation of the technology currently available. One study evaluating gut microbial community structure in relation to adherence to the HEI-2010 showed significant differences between the lowest and highest tertiles of HEI scores (Maskarinec et al., 2019). According to Lampe, several groups of bacteria associated with adherence to the HEI-2010 diet were involved in fiber fermentation. The researchers evaluated a spider plot depicting the 12 component scores of the HEI-2010 (see Figure 2-3) and found that the intake of particular subsets of fruit and vegetables was the major contributor to differences in

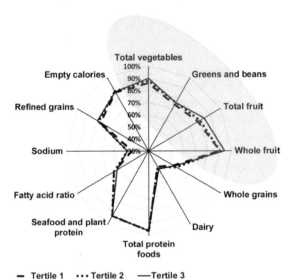

FIGURE 2-3 Spider plot representing the 12 component scores of the Healthy Eating Index-2010 by tertiles of alpha diversity, highlighting fruit and vegetable intake as major contributors to alpha diversity.
SOURCES: Presented by Johanna Lampe on August 15, 2023, from Maskarinec et al., 2019. Reprinted with permission from Elsevier.

the alpha diversity of the microbiome, with little effect being due to refined grains and other components on the plot. Lampe added that other studies have also supported the finding that healthy dietary patterns are associated with an abundance of fiber-fermenting microbes (Peters et al., 2023).

Lampe went on to describe another approach to looking at biomarkers and diet quality—the use of controlled interventions. She cited an analysis comparing the DASH diet against two other diets in a controlled feeding study. The researchers found that multiple metabolites appeared on the metabolomics platform, including many lipid compounds, which were substantially different across diets (Rebholz et al., 2018). Lampe cautioned, however, that taking this analysis to the next level of application to observational studies is complicated and biomarkers cannot necessarily be generalized from a controlled feeding study to the broader food intake of a general population.

Shifting to another approach to biomarker discovery, Lampe discussed work on developing new dietary biomarkers through the Nutrition and Physical Activity Feeding Study. Unlike studies in which all participants consume the same food, the researchers in this study provided each woman with food that resembled her usual diet. The initial step, Lampe explained, was to demonstrate proof of concept and determine whether this study design could elucidate a relationship between serum measures of certain nutrients and the actual intake of those nutrients in the feeding study (Lampe et al., 2017). She reported that robust associations were found between nutrients and their biomarkers, and this finding is now being applied to dietary patterns (Neuhouser et al., 2021). As another example, Lampe referenced a collaboration between researchers studying two different populations. In the Spanish PREDIMED trial, participants' adherence to the Mediterranean diet was associated with a metabolomic signature of 67 metabolites. These metabolites were then shown to independently predict cardiovascular disease risk in the Harvard U.S. Nurses' Health Studies I and II and Health Professionals Follow-up Study (Li et al., 2020).

In summary, Lampe pointed to the variety of -omics approaches that have emerged over the past several decades that can be applied to dietary patterns and diet quality. The most progress, she noted, has been realized in metabolomics biomarkers in blood and urine as objective measures of dietary intake. She added, however, that gaps remain with respect to replication with more ethnically diverse populations, and longitudinal studies examining biomarkers in the context of chronic disease progression.

REVIEW OF THE EVIDENCE ON DIETARY PATTERNS AND CHRONIC DISEASE ACROSS THE LIFESPAN

Edward L. Giovannucci, Harvard University, began by reviewing the three main approaches for evaluating dietary patterns: use of indices or scores based on prior knowledge, empirical analysis based on dietary data, and the hypothesis-oriented approach. For the available indices, he pointed to the frequent overlap among dietary patterns, but he noted that the indices do differ in how they treat certain items. Turning to the empirical method, he explained that it typically involves a principal component analysis. With this method, he observed, there is general concordance in the derived dietary patterns across diverse countries, although some differences exist based on culture or availability of items (e.g., prevalence of sugar-sweetened beverages). Finally, he elaborated on the hypothesis approach, which entails selecting biomarkers and then examining the diet to see what foods predict those biomarkers. He noted that some of the biomarkers studied this way, such as low-density lipoprotein cholesterol, have proven to be strong predictors, but that further studies of this method are needed for it to be more robust. As an example of an empirical or hybrid approach, he shared a study done with different cohorts in which C-peptide and inflammatory markers were selected as biomarkers. Overall, the results showed what might be expected of proinsulinemic and proinflammatory patterns. Giovannucci noted that there is also a fair amount of overlap between these two patterns, which makes sense as inflammation is a determinant of insulin resistance.

Giovannucci went on to state that researchers study dietary patterns for multiple reasons, such as an improved ability to identify additive and synergistic effects of individual nutrients or foods. Moreover, he said, studying an overall dietary pattern inherently accounts for substitution of foods and reduces the problem of confounding seen in many nutritional studies. According to Giovannucci, focusing on individual foods can exaggerate beneficial effects of specific items while ignoring those foods that may have a deleterious effect on health, so defining the overall dietary pattern is more likely to provide a realistic estimate of the potential effect of the diet on chronic disease. The bottom line, he observed, is identifying shared attributes among different dietary patterns and seeing how they relate to major chronic diseases. Giovannucci shared some recent results of a study in this area comparing eight different dietary patterns. The researchers found that the Alternative HEI, the Mediterranean diet, a plant-based diet, a diabetes risk-reduction pattern, and the DASH diet were all strongly protective, being associated with an up to 24 percent reduction in risk of chronic disease (Wang et al., 2023). Giovannucci added that several of the diets were quite similar in their risk reduction.

In conclusion, Giovannucci observed that there are different pathways for disease and that there is clearly much overlap in dietary patterns. He identified three factors involved in predicting disease: the strength of the association between a diet and a particular intermediate, the importance of the intermediate with the specific disease, and the relative importance of the disease. The key message, he suggested, is that dietary patterns represent a useful approach for research and public health messaging, and multiple varied approaches to assessing these patterns have been shown to converge on consistent dietary factors in disease.

DEVELOPMENTAL ORIGINS OF CHRONIC DISEASE AND THE INFLUENCE OF DIET

Robert Waterland, Baylor College of Medicine, highlighted his laboratory's recent discovery that the entire field of epigenetic epidemiology has a major problem affecting its work, and that this problem extends to work toward understanding the developmental origins of health and disease (DOHaD). He shared a magazine cover story from 1999 about how the odds of obesity, cancer, and heart attack are determined when an individual is still in the womb. This phenomenon refers to a paradigm postulating that during critical periods of development, nutrients and other environmental stimuli can affect developmental pathways and have a permanent effect on chronic disease risk. Waterland added that this kind of metabolic imprinting can be thought of as adaptive responses to early nutrition (Waterland and Garza, 1999).

According to Waterland, one potential mechanism explaining the lifelong persistence of metabolic imprinting is epigenetics, defined as the study of mitotically heritable, stable alterations in gene expression potential not caused by changes in DNA sequence. As the best example of this, he cited cell type–specific gene expression potential. Essentially all cells in the human body contain the same DNA (one's entire genome), he elaborated, but different cell types express different subsets of those genes, as established during early development—so some cells become skin cells and others become eye cells, for example. Waterland then framed most of his remarks around an exception to this phenomenon: systemic interindividual epigenetic variation—in which differences are seen among individuals but few differences among different cell types or tissues within each individual.

To understand epigenetic etiology from a DOHaD perspective, Waterland continued, it helps to consider a two-step causal pathway: first, an early environmental exposure during a critical period of development must induce an epigenetic change; then, this change must persist into later life to influence risk of some disease. Waterland described how 20 years ago, in an animal model example, his group demonstrated such a pathway for the first time by showing that methyl donor supplementation of female mice before and during pregnancy permanently increased DNA methylation (an epigenetic mark) at the *agouti viable yellow* locus in their offspring, causing a shift in their coat color toward brown (Waterland and Jirtle, 2003). Motivated by such animal studies, the researchers set out to see whether they could identify metastable epialleles in humans based on their characteristic systemic interindividual variation in DNA methylation. They identified putative metastable epialleles, and through a collaboration in The Gambia found that season of conception (a proxy for maternal nutritional status) influences the establishment of DNA methylation at these loci. Specifically, Waterland elaborated, children conceived in the rainy season tended to have higher methylation at candidate metastable epialleles compared with those conceived in the dry season (Waterland et al., 2010). Another study showed this finding was indeed related to variation in maternal nutritional status around the time of conception (Dominguez-Salas et al., 2014). Essentially, Waterland summarized, early nutrition has an important influence on the establishment of these persistent methylation marks in humans.

With all the collective work in this area from his and other groups, Waterland said it is now clear that these metastable epiallele regions are an obvious place to focus. He explained that testing the second step in the two-step causal pathway—associations among these induced epigenetic changes and risk of later disease—is epigenetic epidemiology. He cautioned, however, that epigenetic epidemiology is much more complicated than genetic epidemiology. He identified one problem as reverse causality—even if epigenetic differences are seen between individuals with and without disease, it can be difficult to determine whether these are a cause or consequence of the disease. According to Waterland, the newest obstacle confronting the field (the "major problem" he referred to in his introduction) is that epigenetic epidemiologists have, for more than a decade, standardized to using Illumina methylation arrays; however, more than 95 percent of the methylation sites interrogated by these arrays show negligible interindividual variation in normal somatic tissue (Gunasekara et al., 2023). Without interindividual variation, he stressed, it is impossible to detect population-level associations (Gunasekara and Waterland, 2019).

Waterland asserted that this problem influences nearly every study in the field, as the Illumina arrays have for more than 10 years been the default tool for epigenetic epidemiology. The problem came to his group's attention following a large screening study in 2019 that identified nearly 10,000 correlated regions of systemic interindividual epigenetic variation (CoRSIVs) (Gunasekara et al., 2019). Waterland explained that metastable epialleles are a subset of CoRSIVs. His group also showed that, although strongly genetically determined, CoRSIVs (not just metastable epialleles) exhibit sensitivity to periconceptional nutrition. Waterland firmly believes that, given the systemic nature of their interindividual variation and their sensitivity to periconceptional environment, a focus on CoRSIVs will greatly improve the ability to detect associations with disease, and called for a fresh start in the field of epigenetic epidemiology.

DISCUSSION

A participant asked about key scientific gaps and areas for improving understanding of the relationship between different food components and dietary patterns and risk of chronic disease. Reedy pointed to opportunities offered by the healthy eating trajectory and how it might be modeled. She noted that historically, the field has looked at this dynamic phenomenon in a static way, and that time-varying models across the life course show promise. Lampe asserted that having enough variation in intake of a food within a study population is critical for understanding that food's impact on risk of disease. "If we don't see a relationship," she asked, "is it because no one is eating a certain food or because they are all eating the same amount?" Giovannucci highlighted the challenge of balancing whether to group items together or study them individually in research, citing the nutritional component differences among many fruits and vegetables. Finally, Waterland offered that it is important to focus on dietary patterns in women before and during early pregnancy, as those choices have the potential to influence, for life, the function of every cell in her child's body.

Another participant emphasized the need to look at diet within the total context of behavioral variables, such as exercise and energy expenditure. Giovannucci pointed to the many overlapping and sometimes redundant pathways involved. Looking at insulin and inflammatory patterns, for example, someone who is inactive and has excess weight tends to also be insulin resistant, so diet is even more important for that individual. Reedy added that it will always be important to embed the HEI or some other pattern within the broader context of other modifiable risk factors. She also highlighted the opportunity to make models that measure dietary patterns nimbler and more nuanced, perhaps by looking upstream and considering how various social determinants of health influence risk factors.

3

Dimensions of Food Choice and Influences on Dietary Patterns

This session, moderated by Alison Brown, National Institutes of Health, began with two speakers providing an overview of inequities in nutrition and health, including opportunities for intervention during the important period of adolescence. Speakers then discussed access to healthy diets globally and the potential to influence food choice through behavioral economics.

INEQUITIES IN NUTRITION AND HEALTH

If one looks at national trends in adult diet quality, said Cindy Leung, Harvard University, one can see modest improvements from 1999 to 2010, but when the data are stratified by socioeconomic status (SES), it is clear that the gains have been made predominantly by those in the highest SES group. Leung asserted that interventions developed to improve diet quality should be universal but ideally should reduce disparities as well. She defined "diet-related health disparities" as "differences in dietary intake, dietary behaviors, and diet patterns in different segments of the population, resulting in poorer diet quality and inferior health outcomes for certain groups and an unequal burden in terms of disease incidence, morbidity, mortality, survival, and quality of life" (Satia, 2009, p. 2).

While individual factors can influence disparities, Leung continued, her remarks would focus on the structural drivers of food insecurity. She defined "food security" as all people at all times having physical and economic access to safe and nutritious foods that meet their dietary needs and food preferences for an active and healthy life. If any of those components are missing, she stated, it will be at the cost of food insecurity. Leung reported that in 2021, the national prevalence of food insecurity in the United States was just over 10 percent, and that some level of insecurity can be found across the country. She shared a map from Feeding America illustrating the breadth of the issue (see Figure 3-1), adding that those at higher risk of food insecurity include households with children, those headed by a single parent, and Black and Hispanic households. She also clarified that while food security and poverty are correlated, they are not the same thing, and families can experience one without the other.

Food insecurity is absolutely a health issue, Leung argued, with documented consequences, such as higher prevalence of diabetes, poor glycemic control and other medication nonadherence for those with diabetes, higher risk of metabolic syndrome, greater odds of inflammation, and higher prevalence of hypertension. She added that those who experience food insecurity also typically have lower scores for the healthy diet patterns discussed previously (see Chapter 2). The more severe the food insecurity experienced by a family or person, the worse their diet quality is, she noted. When her team studied which specific aspects of diet were affected, they were surprised to find that not just certain food groups but all dietary

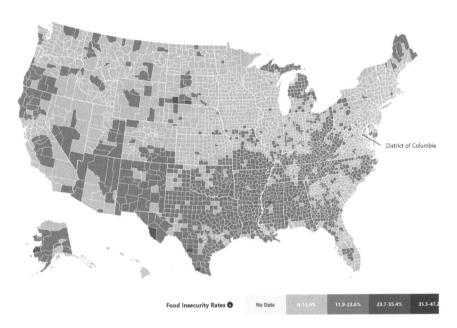

FIGURE 3-1 Food insecurity among the overall (all ages) population in the United States.
SOURCES: Presented by Cindy Leung on August 15, 2023, from Gundersen et al., 2023. Reprinted with permission from Feeding America.

components, as defined by the Prime Diet Quality Score 30-day screener, were in the adverse direction (Wolfson et al., 2022). To learn more about these associations, the researchers conducted qualitative research in the San Francisco Bay Area, asking families which factors affected their ability to feed their children the food they wanted to eat. Key themes emerged from this work, she reported, including how the environment nudges people toward foods that do not support health, how food insecurity requires additional cognitive and physical effort, and how food insecurity serves as a source of toxic stress. Once these factors are understood, Leung argued, interventions can then be developed. She acknowledged the strong network of federal food programs that serve millions of low-income families, allowing them better access to nutritious food, but she also posited that perhaps these programs are not enough.

When the COVID-19 pandemic began, Leung said, she was surprised that food insecurity levels did not spike as early studies had indicated (Wolfson and Leung, 2020). As one of the main reasons for this, she pointed to active mobilizing of the Supplemental Nutrition Assistance Program (SNAP), including an increase in the minimum benefit level, additional administrative support, and an online purchasing pilot. To improve the program even further, SNAP participants surveyed by her team suggested increasing the minimum benefit to $30/month, increasing distribution frequency to biweekly, and subsidizing online grocery delivery fees (Wolfson et al., 2021). Nearly 90 percent of their survey respondents wanted extra money to be used for fruits and vegetables, Leung added, noting that a bill addressing this prospect—the Hot Foods Act[1]—is currently under consideration.

Leung continued by suggesting that, while food assistance programs are critical to ensuring food security, it may be time to look beyond traditional federal programs. From the Household Pulse Survey, conducted during the COVID-19 pandemic, she elaborated, it became clear that when families receive stimulus checks and child tax credits, food insufficiency (a proxy for food insecurity) can be reduced. According to Leung, then, there is an opportunity beyond SNAP to think about economic programs as interventions, which would provide a more robust suite of food and economic policies to help eliminate food insecurity.

Tashara M. Leak, Cornell University, stressed the potential to establish healthful dietary behaviors, partly because in adolescence, individuals start to have more autonomy and purchasing power in making food choices. In low-income households and those that have been racially and ethnically minoritized, she elaborated, adolescents are often doing the grocery

---

[1] Hot Foods Act, S. 2258, H.R. 3519.

shopping and cooking for the entire family; they may be thought of as children but should be recognized as functioning like adults.

Leak observed that obesity is more prevalent in adolescents than in younger children and is linked to an increased risk of prediabetes in adulthood. Additionally, this risk is not evenly distributed, as there are income and racial disparities in the prevalence of prediabetes nationally (Liu et al., 2022). Leak emphasized the importance of the language used to talk to parents about this issue, as illustrated by her experience trying to convince families that they needed to make changes in their children's diet because of obesity concerns. She encountered difficulties because of cultural norms around body size and body image, as well as parents' competing concerns, such as just putting food on the table or finding dependable work. Explaining the linkages between obesity and prediabetes, however, is much more likely to motivate parents to make changes to ensure that their children stay healthy.

Another factor to consider in the diet of adolescents, given their autonomy, is snacking, said Leak. She reported that 23 percent of daily energy intake among U.S. adolescents comes from snacks, and on a given day, 73 percent of adolescents consume items from the snacks and sweets category, such as chips and cookies (Gangrade et al., 2021). Not surprisingly, Leak added, there are even disparities in snacking behavior, such that adolescents from low-income homes consume more added sugar and less whole grains, fruit, and fiber compared with their peers from higher-income homes. She explained that many adolescents face structural barriers—such as an abundance of corner stores offering options that are less healthy but often more expensive—that prevent them from making healthier choices in urban environments. Yet, she pointed out, this is where many adolescents go to purchase snacks. Likewise, between 2006 and 2018, the number of quick-service restaurants located near public schools in urban communities increased from 25 to 34 percent (Olarte et al., 2023), creating even more opportunities for less healthy snacking.

Leak next shared an equity-oriented obesity prevention action framework, with four target areas (Kumanyika, 2019): increasing healthy options through the built environment; reducing deterrents to healthy eating; building on community capacity; focusing on sustainability; and improving social and economic resources.

Leak then shared examples of interventions in schools, clinical settings, and community centers aimed at putting this framework into action. Referring to the previous observation about parents having competing interests, she acknowledged that getting them invested in their children's nutrition can be difficult. She noted that when parents are worried about their children going hungry or their electricity being shut off, they may consider it an unaffordable privilege to pay attention to foods' nutritional content. She also highlighted the importance of not abandoning cultural food norms in an effort to eat healthy, which can further add to disparities. Her programs focus on plant-based dishes in various cuisines and connect nutrition education with culinary education so that adolescents can understand how to make healthy foods in their own home.

For the long term, Leak emphasized the importance of dissemination and implementation of equity-oriented obesity preventing interventions across all settings to promote the interventions' sustainability. She pointed to opportunities through 4-H partnerships, work on policy with local governments and school boards, collaborations with health systems to help physicians think outside the box in seeking to help adolescents, and partnerships with community organizations and health departments to advance equity efforts in academic infrastructures to address pressing societal issues.

DISCUSSION

Questions and discussions centered around the social and cultural factors related to dietary behavior. Regarding social factors, Leak said it will be critical to collaborate across disciplines and sectors and to acknowledge other components of family life that may prevent families from thinking about nutrition. Simultaneously, she asserted, changes must be made at the policy level. Leung agreed, noting that food insecurity is correlated with the social determinants of health, so it can feel overwhelming to move the needle. She stressed, however, that structural drivers of food insecurity must be addressed. Leung observed that food insecurity is rooted in poverty, structural racism, and many systemic inequities. She added that the field needs to move away from the message that everyone needs to follow the Mediterranean diet to be healthy; rather, all cultures and ethnic groups have respective dietary patterns that can fit within national guidelines. Therefore, she suggested, training dietitians to have sensitivity and understanding when working with different populations and aligning the guidelines with each family's cultural background can be significant in sustaining the adoption of a healthy diet.

FOOD CHOICE AND ACCESS TO HEALTHY DIETS

Understanding of food choice and dietary patterns in the United States can be informed by data on access to healthy diets worldwide, began William Masters, Tufts University. In economics, he continued, preferences are inferred from observed choices, with price and income elasticities obtained through demand system estimation. He went on to explain that since 2018, new studies have extended the economics toolkit using nutritional data so that analysts can measure a population's access to a healthy diet compared with what they actually consume. This new work enables analysts to measure how much it would cost to meet a population's health needs and whether a healthy diet is affordable using locally available foods. The method is used both within individual countries and globally to monitor change in the number of people who cannot afford a healthy diet, for which the latest estimate from the United Nations was 3.1 billion people worldwide.

The purpose of measuring access to a healthy diet, Masters continued, is to diagnose why unhealthy diets are consumed and identify one of three kinds of remedies. First, when items are unavailable or local prices are high for even the least expensive version of a healthy diet, interventions are needed to improve the supply of suitable items in the food groups identified as unusually expensive or unavailable. At other places and times, availability and prices may be normal, but households have insufficient income to afford enough of even the least expensive items in all the food groups needed for health. In those cases, achieving a healthy dietary pattern is possible only with nutrition assistance. Third, a population may face normal prices and have sufficient income, but the items needed for a healthy diet are displaced by other foods.

Masters explained that this new method is being applied globally to measure diet costs using computer models to identify the items that are lowest cost and locally available in sufficient quantities to meet each country's dietary guidelines. This global monitoring uses a composite Healthy Diet Basket (HDB) based on commonalities among all countries' guidelines, including the *Dietary Guidelines for Americans* (DGA).[2] One key aspect of these modeled benchmark diets, Masters observed, is that they use retail item prices; for consumers, the overwhelming contributor to the cost of a food is not its ingredients but its production and distribution—an observation that is especially relevant for half of consumer spending on food away from home. He also highlighted variation over time in food prices, the most severe spikes occurring in wholesale prices (see Figure 3-2), noting that these spikes, exemplified by the high inflation seen during the COVID-19 recovery period, can result in food crises. Yet even when food prices are low, he stressed, many people cannot afford healthy diets.

Masters described new work focused on the lowest-cost diets that meet dietary guidelines, allowing measurement of access to and affordability of sufficiently nutritious food and distinguishing among three possible causes of poor diet quality: the high cost of nutritious foods, insufficient income to acquire them, and food choice among affordable items. In its 2020 *Annual State of Food Security and Nutrition Report*, the Food and Agriculture

---

[2] HDB is a globally relevant dietary standard that reflects the common elements of most national food-based dietary guidelines (Herforth et al., 2022).

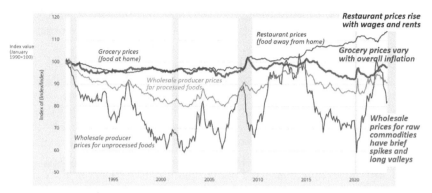

FIGURE 3-2 Consumer prices for groceries and restaurant meals vs. wholesale costs, January 1990–June 2023.
SOURCES: Presented by William Masters on August 15, 2023, data from U.S. Bureau of Labor Statistics (data from August 5, 2023).

Organization of the United Nations included, for the first time, the cost of recommended diets that met 10 different dietary guidelines around the world. Masters shared the costs of the least expensive food items globally. In 2017, for example, the average cost for just the daily energy needed to meet caloric needs was $0.83/day; for the least expensive diet for nutrient adequacy was $2.46/day; and for a healthy diet meeting national dietary guidelines was $3.31/day. This latter diet includes 11 distinct items in six food groups, and while there are commonalities across countries, each country will have a different mix of 11 items that reach the HDB targets for balance based on what is available and widely consumed in that country.

Looking at the cost and affordability of these diets, Masters continued, the findings were stunning even for the lowest-cost diet meeting energy sufficiency. His group found that around 3 billion people worldwide—essentially 40 percent of the global population—cannot afford even this minimalist HDB for energy sufficiency, a point made earlier by Leak. This is the first ability to distinguish between lack of affordability and choice from among affordable options. Most of the unaffordability, Masters elaborated, was found to be due to low incomes, so that healthier diets would require higher earnings, whereas in the United States and other high-income countries, the cause of poor diet quality is food choice among affordable options.

Masters went on to observe that healthy diets being affordable does not mean people are food secure, as these concepts measure different things. He explained that "food insecurity," as currently measured, means survey respondents had run out of money to buy their usual diet at least once over the previous year. Thus while food insecurity is important, it refers to usual diets consumed and not a dietary pattern that would meet the DGA or other dietary guidelines, he said. Using modeled diets to calculate what it would cost to meet the DGA, Masters elaborated, reveals whether those usual diets are of low nutritional quality because prices are high, in which case there is an opportunity to intervene on the supply side to lower costs. Thus when costs are normal but incomes are low, intervention with income assistance can provide support. Masters contrasted this situation with one in which people have adequate income to buy the food needed for a healthy diet, but those foods are displaced by unhealthy foods. Masters concluded by listing several potential areas for intervention, including time use, cost of meal preparation, identifying items with the most potential to improve diets, and identifying people who need higher incomes to afford a healthy diet.

IMPROVING HEALTH THROUGH BEHAVIORAL ECONOMICS

It is understood that food is central to health outcomes, began Kevin Volpp, University of Pennsylvania, but fewer than 1 in 10 Americans meet recommendations for the consumption of fruits and vegetables. He added that at the same time, more than 9 in 10 have excess sodium intake, and only 2 percent meet targets for whole grains. He focused his remarks on the behavioral challenges preventing people from eating healthy food.

Volpp stressed the importance of recognizing that rationality can inadequately describe behavior change. People have difficulty making trade-offs between the present and the future, he observed, and decades of research in behavioral economics have shown that the mind has multiple types of behavioral reflexes. He noted that these reflexes are often used to bypass cognition because not every single decision can be weighed by risk, benefit, and probabilities of potential outcomes. He offered three implications for thinking about interventions, recommending consideration of approaches that are based on choice architecture and financial and social incentives instead of just providing information to consumers.

First, Volpp continued, presenting different options and changing default choices can increase the likelihood that people will choose healthy items; examples include providing "opt-out" rather than "opt-in" defaults for programs or listing healthier choices first. He noted that this approach was modeled with a population of people with poorly controlled diabetes who were offered a free program for wireless monitoring at home. One group was offered the opt-in option, while the other was told they were automatically enrolled unless they did not want to be. The study showed that this simple reframing of the invitation tripled enrollment rates, said Volpp; patient engagement and improvements in patient A1C (blood glucose) showed a similar pattern (Aysola et al., 2018). According to Volpp, this research showed not only that low enrollment rates can be improved by framing enrollment as a default for eligible patients, but also that, where possible, choice architecture can be used to help guide the choice of healthy foods, and that simply shifting some of the default settings in the health record can help clinicians refer more patients to such interventions.

As a second implication, Volpp observed that financial incentives can be highly effective, but their effectiveness depends on design. For example, he continued, a tax on sugary beverages can result in decreased consumption of less healthy choices. He cited a study in Philadelphia showing that a 1.5 cent per ounce tax on sugar-sweetened beverages was associated with a 38 percent net decrease in their consumption (Roberto et al., 2019). Globally, he added, a 10 percent increase in price decreases consumption of such beverages by about 8 percent (Chaloupka et al., 2019). Conversely, he explained, subsidizing healthy foods has not been shown to increase their consumption by much. Part of the challenge here is the asymmetry of gains and losses, he elaborated: if people are not buying healthy foods regularly, they may not pay enough attention to them to notice sales or discounts. Additionally, he pointed out, research in psychology has found that the utility of a dollar lost is roughly twice the utility of a dollar gained, which he said helps explain why price increases have a greater effect than price decreases on utilization. Volpp pointed out that a similar phenomenon is seen in the health system with copayments: when they are raised, health care utilization drops, but when they are lowered, health care utilization does not increase very much. Thus, he stressed, it is important to think critically about the behavioral mechanisms involved and systematically test ways to tap into them. Importantly, he said, the incentives do not need to be large to work, but they need to be immediate, salient, and presented in a way that is easy to understand.

Lastly, Volpp referred to the launching of the American Heart Association's (AHA's) Food Is Medicine initiative, funded by the Rockefeller Foundation and inaugural partner Kroger, with a goal of building evidence for scaling these programs more widely. He noted that while lifestyle interventions can be very effective, they are not always covered by insurance to the same extent as pharmaceuticals, which makes them difficult to sustain. Volpp cited a 2002 study showing a lower incidence of diabetes for participants in the Diabetes Prevention Program compared with those on the drug metformin (Diabetes Prevention Program Research Group, 2002); although all insurers covered metformin, it took another 12–14 years for them to cover the Diabetes Prevention Program. Volpp emphasized the double standard involved, in that lifestyle interventions are often covered only if they yield short-term savings, whereas medications are covered if found by the U.S. Food and Drug Administration to be safe and effective regardless of their cost-effectiveness.

Volpp acknowledged that important evidence on which to build has been gleaned from the Special Supplemental Nutrition Program for Women,

Infants, and Children; medically tailored meals; and other available programs; however, he argued, much remains to be learned in terms of intensity, duration, delivery, and engagement. He described a research planning group of national experts—with expertise in areas ranging from food as medicine, to clinical trial design, to cost-effectiveness, to behavioral science—that has been charged with thinking about ways to ensure that the AHA initiative will have a large impact. He noted that one of the focal points for the AHA program is human-centered design, focused on better understanding current behavior and rapidly iterating the aspects of the program.

Volpp reported that a cooperative studies model for accelerating learning is being developed. "We want to be able to learn from one another as rapidly as possible," he explained, "and not wait until the end of each study to find out what happened." Volpp's group hopes to maximize learning across pilot sites and use automated trial platforms to facilitate replicating and scaling efforts. The group is just finishing the planning phase for the 10-year initiative, he added, and next will be looking to derisk the larger-scale trials and conduct rapid-cycle testing of feasibility, efficacy, and the like. Overall, he concluded, this initiative will be focused on improving health equity and building programs to be scaled.

DISCUSSION

Participants and speakers highlighted different perspectives on making some of the choices connected to food. Volpp, for example, referred to decision fatigue for those with lower incomes, stating that it is tied to the broader issue of scarcity. Individuals living in poverty are essentially burdened by the taxing of their cognitive bandwidth, and it is difficult to make decisions when one is constantly in cognitive overload. According to Volpp, this is another reason to think deliberately about designing solutions that make it easier to choose healthy foods. From an agricultural perspective, a participant asked if the right foods were being produced. Masters stressed that too little land and resources are devoted to producing fruits, vegetables, and fish. He suggested making land use more inclusive, devising more jobs for people, and creating a smaller climate footprint.

Another participant asked about the cost of housing as context. Masters noted that, when one considers financial precarity, food insecurity, and adverse living conditions, it is clear that the lack of housing for people in the United States is central to structural deprivation. Zoning restrictions add challenges to this deprivation, he pointed out, as do transportation and access to employment. He asserted that all these issues of livelihood and security underlie the overarching challenge of food insecurity.

4

Role of Industry and
Consumer Perspectives

The speakers in the next session, moderated by Alison Brown, National Institutes of Health, began by reviewing the challenges consumers face in choosing healthy diets. Speakers then described varying industry perspectives on how to promote these healthy behaviors and actions being taken to facilitate that process, thus looking to the future for sustainability and next-generation programming.

NEUROPHYSIOLOGY OF CONSUMER CHOICE

Marco A. Palma, Texas A&M University, reviewed the neurophysiology of consumer food choice, beginning with an evolutionary biology trip back to the time when humans were hunters and gatherers and spent most of their energy securing food for survival. During that time, he explained, the brain provided rewards in ways that are similar to reward responses for highly addictive substances today. Now, he said, humans typically spend much less time foraging and securing food, making it relatively cheaper and easier to obtain; however, the brain's evolution has not kept pace with advances in agriculture, and humans still live in a world that rewards them anatomically for finding and consuming sugar-dense food. When humans face these urges, he added, there is a connection between the reward system and the brain circuitry—particularly in the regions related to self-control—that determines enjoyment of food.

Palma went on to review evidence from neuroeconomics showing that the brain regions activated when people see words like "healthy eating" are different from those activated by more emotionally driven, hedonic messages related to tasty food. But not everyone, he observed, experiences the same self-control urges. Palma referred to two predominant and seemingly contradictory theories proposed to explain self-control. One theory suggests that self-control is like a snowball: the more one engages in an activity, the more motivation is generated, and the greater is the likelihood of exerting self-control in the same or unrelated activities. The second theory says self-control is a finite resource, and once people have run out of it, they are unable to access and use it. Palma proposed, however, that these are not two different theories but parts of the same unified theory that are missing a compliance measure to link them. Essentially, he elaborated, the initial act of self-control enhances subsequent acts, but once self-control is overdone or drastic measures are taken, it becomes overwhelmingly difficult to continue to exercise restraint, and people can set themselves up to fail by trying to do too much (Palma et al., 2018).

As a closing example, Palma shared a study in which consumers were given wine to taste from two different bottles; the wine in both bottles was identical except for the price tag. Participants' brain activity was then measured through functional magnetic resonance imaging. The researchers found that the medial orbitofrontal cortex, a region of the brain associated with pleasure, was activated more with the expensive bottle of wine than with the lower-priced bottle (Plassmann et al., 2008). Palma explained that this finding is crucial because it illustrates the importance of nonphysical attributes of foods and their critical role in determining how much pleasure consumers derive from eating them.

INSTACART

Beatrice Abiero, Instacart, discussed how the grocery technology company partners with more than 1,400 retailers across the United States and Canada to provide access to grocery delivery for more than 95 percent of households. Over the past decade, she said, Instacart has worked at the intersection of food and people, which also means it intersects with health, and the company is rethinking how it can become more of a health enablement platform. She reported that last year the company launched Instacart Health with the goal of expanding access to nutritious food and delivering healthy outcomes. She described the three pillars of the program: improving nutrition security, making healthy choices easier, and scaling food-as-medicine programs. Abiero highlighted Fresh Funds, which allows any entity, including hospitals or researchers, to produce category-restricted stipends and related food-as-medicine programs online. A second initiative is Virtual Storefronts, which allows entities to provide a branded, customized experience to show different dietary regimens.

Given Instacart's technology and reach across the continent, Abiero continued, it is uniquely positioned for research opportunities and can provide infrastructure to programs. For example, Instacart partnered with the University of Kentucky and No Kid Hungry to conduct a study aimed at better understanding the impact of online groceries and their delivery for families on tight budgets. Following extensive analysis of receipts and survey data, Abiero reported, the study found that individuals were able to stretch their food budgets, decrease stigma, and save time when grocery shopping online. For those who shopped online and received additional guidance in navigating the online environment, an average increase of nearly $7 was spent on fruit and vegetable purchases. Abiero concluded by stating that collaborations will focus on empowering patients to navigate the food system with tools at their fingertips, integrating recipes, and supporting the American Heart Association's Food Is Medicine initiative. These studies shape how Instacart centers the user experience, she explained, and she is excited to continue working with researchers to empower consumers to improve their health.

KELLOGG COMPANY

Sarah Ludmer, Kellogg Company, shared the company's plan to give "better days" to 3 million people by the end of 2030 by approaching the goal in four intersecting ways: sustainability; well-being; hunger; and equity, diversity, and inclusion. Over the past 20 years, she said, Kellogg has focused on making food healthier by increasing such components as whole grains and fiber while also reducing "negative ingredients," such as sodium and sugar. She argued, however, that a shift is needed in how to provide equitable food access more broadly and in how "nourishing" is defined. In 2016, for example, Kellogg petitioned the U.S. Food and Drug Administration (FDA) to increase the amount of vitamin D allowed in cereals. At the end of 2022, this request was approved, and all manufacturers can now offer increased vitamin D levels in their foods. Ludmer emphasized the importance of focusing on positive nutrients and on eating more healthy foods, saying that this focus can be more impactful than just avoiding the intake of unhealthy foods. She pointed to research showing that eating more healthy foods, such as whole grains, fruits, vegetables, and nuts, had a greater impact on overall mortality than did reducing the intake of unhealthy foods. She noted, however, that studies also have shown that high intakes of sodium have a direct impact on mortality, so she emphasized that it is important to think about the overall picture of health and diet.

According to Ludmer, cereal is a food that repeatedly plays a role in the intake of different nutrients for many Americans. She observed that cereal eaters are typically found to have higher intakes of the shortfall nutrients (such as iron and folate) and higher overall scores on the Healthy Eating Index (Zhu et al., 2022); moreover, they do not have higher intakes of added sugar and have less intake of sodium and saturated fat than those who do not eat cereal. Taking a broader view, Ludmer characterized the Special Supplemental Nutrition Program for Women, Infants, and Children (WIC) as the first food-as-medicine program. It emphasizes positive food and nutrients first with health outcomes in mind, she said, while including foods that complement one another and provide diversity in the diet. Although she acknowledged that not all the foods in the WIC program may meet the proposed FDA definition of healthy, she asserted that they offer important nutritional advantages and have shown remarkable health outcomes for participants.

In closing, Ludmer highlighted Kellogg's focus on driving increased redemption within the WIC program, as currently only 60 percent of people redeem their WIC cereal dollars. She stressed that Kellogg is committed to continuing to advocate for positive nudges toward healthy foods.

SEASON HEALTH

Josh Hix, Season Health, characterized his company as a food-as-medicine platform, offering three primary interventions to help drive health outcomes: clinical services, a food marketplace, and benefit assistance. Changing the food environment digitally around a consumer can be impactful, he maintained, and he shared health outcomes based on Medicaid data showing positive changes in markers such as hemoglobin A1C (blood glucose) levels, body mass index, and blood pressure in just 90 days by putting a consumer-grade intervention in front of the patients or the health plan member. He observed that, taken together, the above three interventions map to comments by previous speakers on choice architecture, changing the food environment, and making the healthy choice the obvious choice.

Elaborating on the three Season Health interventions, Hix explained that the company's virtual clinic offers engagement with registered dietitians for support; the marketplace offers diverse food options and medically tailored meals; and the benefits bank works with food credits, waivers, and program benefits such as the Supplemental Nutrition Assistance Program (SNAP) and WIC so that participants can make the most of their available funding to change their dietary behaviors. He noted that while Season Health is a for-profit business, the only way it gets paid is by driving health outcomes, and it does not monetize any of the food options provided. He added that the company's focus is on populations already living with chronic disease, but he is hopeful that in several years, this model will also be scaled and reimbursed for preventive care in healthier populations.

DISCUSSION

Speakers and participants discussed the importance of the cultural appropriateness of foods, choice architecture, and how labels can influence consumer decision making. Addressing consumer testing and cultural appropriateness of foods, Hix replied that Season Health pairs members with a dietitian for culinary and nutrition education. He explained that the company emphasizes the right alignment and incentives with health plans to offer the widest possible variety, and in some locations that have the necessary density of health plans, it establishes local kitchens and suppliers, contingent on a threshold density of health plan members who have the funds, typically sponsored through a combination of public benefits such as SNAP and WIC and health plan benefits, to support this model. In this way, he added, people from the community are most likely preparing the food, which may be a healthier version of a local or cultural favorite. The company also partners with local kitchens and community-based organizations to give members an appropriate amount of choice.

Another participant asked for suggestions on how to make the healthy choice the easy choice. Palma replied that consumers tend to perceive a trade-off between health and taste in food, so food labels need to balance the two. He noted that there is limited "real estate" on a food label, so advertising experts must decide how much of that space should be used to promote the healthfulness of products and how much to say that the food is tasty. Ludmer echoed Palma, saying that when people are told that a product is good for them, it often does not sell. She suggested working with retailers to promote items that can easily be used to build a healthy meal so the consumer does not have to think about what to make and which items are needed for each meal.

Abiero identified several touch points that can be used to influence the consumer in partnership with input from health experts, such as the use of tags on groceries highlighting low sodium or low sugar content. Hix noted that Season Health designs nudges based on patients' needs. For example, patients with kidney disease see white bread by design, whereas patients with diabetes see whole-grain bread as their option. At the same time, he explained, the platform tries to ensure that it is offering numerous options that account for the preferences of both patients and their families or members of their household.

Finally, a question was raised about the changes taking place with food labels, whether products can be called healthy or certain nutrients can be highlighted. Ludmer said that Kellogg is advocating for front-of-package systems but that this approach has seen limited success in other countries. She noted further that the positive attributes of a food are difficult to get across on a label. Palma added that people navigate through the grocery store very quickly, and eye-tracking research has shown they do not spend much time looking at labels; instead, they often go to aisles where they know familiar items are located. Finally, Abiero called attention to a point made by previous speakers that the discussion can at times still focus on rating individual products instead of assessing overall diet quality or patterns. To advance progress, she argued, more attention is needed on the dynamic elements of the dietary patterns of individuals.

5

Lessons Learned and Translating Solutions for the Future

In the final session of the workshop, moderated by Fang Fang Zhang, Tufts University, speakers reviewed interventions conducted by various stakeholders to improve the food environments for consumers and populations of different ages. They also highlighted the work of community-based organizations and their role in influencing food infrastructure, as well as food policy. Finally, speakers discussed legal and policy challenges and opportunities for further improving access to healthy foods and health outcomes.

IMPROVING THE HEALTHFULNESS OF FOOD ENVIRONMENTS

Speakers on this topic highlighted work with corner stores and grocery retailers in Minnesota, lessons learned from research in Baltimore, and opportunities for positioning families to succeed by engaging health care providers more systematically.

Improving Access to Healthy Options

Melissa Laska, University of Minnesota, began by explaining that her work builds on the premise that not all Americans have equal access to healthy food—something that has been known for quite some time. Disparities are clearly cut across race, ethnicity, and income, she observed, and many communities lack access to retail food outlets where they can buy a range of healthy foods at reasonable prices. One of the first solutions tried, Laska continued, was to build new supermarkets in those communities, but while job creation and new infrastructure came from these initiatives, the research findings were, in her words, underwhelming. Improvements in dietary patterns among the residents living in these communities were not apparent, Laska elaborated; this likely resulted, in part, from overlooking the numerous smaller food stores that play a key role in many communities. She described these small venues, such as bodegas and corner stores, as trusted retailers having numerous touch points with residents. She noted, for example, that one in three customers surveyed when exiting small food stores in Minneapolis and St. Paul, Minnesota, reported that they shop in that store every day. More than 75 percent reported that they shop in the store at least once a week, she added, which is often enough to offer an opportunity for intervention. Laska acknowledged, however, that there are also challenges involved in working with small food stores, as many of these retailers have not built their business model to account for perishable foods, so they face infrastructure limitations and procurement issues in dealing with these foods.

Efforts targeting these stores to promote the availability of healthy foods began around 15 years ago, said Laska, with technical assistance being provided to small food stores, especially for supplying produce. She noted that there was a great deal of both excitement and success in this first wave of work. Research showed changes in customers' knowledge and attitudes and yielded mixed evidence with regard to changes in purchasing and sales, but implementation challenges impeded further improvements. As one key challenge, however, Laska identified the scalability of implementation, which was highly time and effort intensive. Sustainability issues became clearer over time as well, she added, as effects could be seen during the acute intervention phase in stores, but once that phase had ended, there was often a return to baseline.

Laska shared an example from Minnesota, where there was a very active corner store program. Discussion at the time was focused on policy levers for grocers and business licenses and how to incentivize participation and leverage the opportunity offered by these small stores throughout the city of Minneapolis. In 2014, Laska continued, the Minneapolis Staple Foods ordinance went into effect, mandating that stores stock minimum quantities of certain healthy staple foods. She noted, however, that following a 5-year study of the ordinance's implementation, researchers found very small changes in these stores, with no consistent improvements in the nutritional quality of purchases compared with nearby St. Paul, which did not have this ordinance (see Figure 5-1).

Reflecting on this study and the findings reported in other literature on the subject, Laska said her group has had time to think about what direction to take next. She cited a 2022 review looking at retailer strategies that have been tried and tested across heterogeneous supermarket environments, which found mixed results with regard to changes in sales, purchasing,

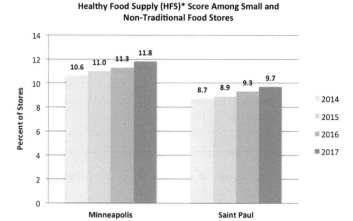

FIGURE 5-1 Healthy Food Supply (HFS) score among small and nontraditional food stores.
NOTE: The HFS score is a measure of the overall healthfulness of store offerings. The level of change is seen to be similar in Minneapolis and St. Paul stores.
SOURCES: Presented by Melissa Laska on August 16, 2023, data from Caspi et al., 2020, and Laska et al., 2019.

and dietary outcomes (Wolgast et al., 2022). One of the more rigorously tested strategies in food stores is nutrition scoring, she noted, whereby shelf tags have quantified labels showing how healthy a product is—a strategy implemented primarily in larger-format stores, and one that requires large-scale implementation across product categories. Laska stressed that ultimately, industry often has control over the store environment and product placement. In talking with store owners, Laska and colleagues have found notable evidence of formal and informal agreements with distributors and food manufacturers that include benefits to the retailer, such as free displays and signage to promote specific products. In exchange, the retailer gives control of placement and price back to the industry. She closed with a call to better understand the scope of these arrangements so as to advance in-store research in a meaningful way.

A Focus on Infants and Children

As a Washington, DC, community pediatrician at Children's National Hospital, Kofi D. Essel, now primarily director of food as medicine at Elevance Health, incorporates nutrition information in his guidance and counseling for patients and families. He acknowledged, however, that this was not always his practice. He related an incident that took place following his interaction with a family and their 4-month-old baby, when he realized that neither he, his colleagues, nor his physician supervisors were equipped to talk to this family about infant feeding and child nutrition. Essel noted that this realization aligns with the literature, which shows that 71 percent of medical schools do not provide the recommended minimum 25 hours of baseline nutrition education, with a third not providing even half that amount (Adams et al., 2015). Overall, he added, even fellows and attending physicians later in their careers did not feel confident in having these discussions with families around nutrition and diet-related chronic disease. While recognizing that physicians do not need to become dietitians, Essel stated his belief that they should feel comfortable enough with the subject to support families with meaningful and unharmful dietary advice. He also expressed his belief that pediatricians should be comfortable providing nutrition support in the first 1,000 days of a child's life, which in his view is often a missed opportunity to prepare the child and the family for success later in life. He added that if one waits until the child is older to provide this support, the child is often already a picky eater and has established other challenging habits and patterns.

The difficulty of understanding the best ways to feed young children is compounded when families experience food insecurity, Essel continued. He noted that food insecurity is often triggered when a family experiences a sudden financial hardship. The food budget is affected because it can easily fluctuate, he elaborated, leading to anxiety around meal acquisition and the quality of food, with diets becoming monotonous in turn, and ultimately the amount of food consumed by every member in the household declining. Essel characterized food insecurity in American households as ubiquitous and quite pervasive, but often invisible, so that clinicians are frequently surprised by how pervasive it is when they ask screening questions. Considering the hierarchy of food needs, he observed, just having enough food to feed the family is the most critical concern for many people who experience food insecurity. Essel stressed further that, although the goal of diversifying a child's diet revolves around offering a variety of foods, there is a good chance that families experiencing food insecurity will be unable to do so because they are worried about wasting money and food. He added that parents enjoy seeing their children happy, so offering foods they know a child already likes makes them feel good, too, and slowly habits are formed around that diet. Essel maintained that infants eventually should eat what adults are eating, but he pointed out that most adults do not eat enough fruits and vegetables and have poor-quality diets overall, thereby perpetuating a cycle that leads to diet-related diseases, a problem that is exacerbated in households experiencing food insecurity.

To address this issue, in 2016, Essel's health system began screening all children at Children's National Hospital for food insecurity. Initially, the parents would be given a list of resources, but often they were not useful for families. Accordingly, Essel said, a clinical community partnership called

FLiP, the Family Lifestyle Program, was created. This program brought together Children's National Hospital, the American Heart Association, and the Young Men's Christian Association of Metropolitan Washington, with a focus on healthy families and communities, addressing food and nutrition security and diet-related chronic disease through a family-centered lens. FLiP included a food-as-medicine program, with a primary emphasis on produce prescriptions, which involved introducing access to fresh, frozen, or canned produce through vouchers or direct delivery for families. Essel's group was especially interested in using the program as an intervention to support the health of young children in their first 1,000 days.

Essel described FLiPRx, the company's produce prescription initiative, a pilot project that involved delivering fresh produce from local farms every other week for 1 year to families who were experiencing food insecurity and those at risk for diet-related disease. FLiPRx also included a variety of nutrition education tools, including community cooking classes. Essel shared some qualitative results of this family pilot project. Fruit and vegetable intake increased, and families reported that they were able to try new foods without worrying about waste, had greater purchasing power, and could better diversify their diet.

In summary, Essel emphasized the importance of understanding that food-insecure households place young children in a stressed feeding environment and typically have poorer diet quality. He added that caregivers need the support of being connected to resources that allow them to expand the children's dietary options without worrying about wasting what is left uneaten. Finally, Essel argued that such interventions not only help improve the quality of food intake for families, but also offer the kind of multifaceted approach that is necessary for building partnerships, designing focus groups, and creating materials in different languages to reach a wide range of groups in need.

Lessons Learned from Food Environments in Baltimore

Joel Gittelsohn, Johns Hopkins University, highlighted his work in Baltimore to improve the food environment, calling attention to a map demonstrating that 20–25 percent of residents live in Healthy Food Priority Areas (previously called "food deserts"). Those areas not only lack access to healthy food, he pointed out, but have an abundance of unhealthy food resources. He added that the median income is below 185 percent of the federal poverty level, and there is limited access to personal vehicles.

According to Gittelsohn, the food environment in Baltimore is large and complex, with numerous public markets, food pantries, supermarkets, convenience stores, and many more retailers, making it difficult to know how to prioritize his group's efforts. The group developed four main approaches: changing the availability of healthy options; changing the availability of unhealthy options; manipulating prices; and addressing location, in terms of both the ability to get to a store and placement of foods within the store. Gittelsohn shared research conducted between 2000 and 2018, noting that most interventions targeted the provider/seller and consumer levels, with some focusing on suppliers such as food banks and wholesalers, but that none of the work touched on policies. Previous studies found that food environment interventions can be effective in addressing key risk behaviors for chronic disease in disadvantaged communities, he acknowledged, by improving access, increasing consumption of healthy foods, and sometimes impacting obesity. His group, however, recognized the importance of multifaceted efforts, integrating educational, access, and policy approaches whenever possible, while emphasizing community engagement at every level.

Describing his group's current work, Gittelsohn shared five lessons learned, presented in Box 5-1. In closing, he observed that his group has taken 20 years to develop and test solutions for improving the food environment, and that such efforts require both capacity and experience.

BOX 5-1
Lessons from Food Environment Research in Baltimore

1. **Invest heavily in formative research (i.e., mixed methods; triangulation; emergent, flexible design).** Relying on a few focus groups will not be sufficient to secure the multiple perspectives and triangulation needed to understand the whole picture. There is often a disconnect between retailers and consumers, so communication linkages are critical to improving the food environment.
2. **Engage with communities for the long term.** This is not a new lesson, but it can be difficult to do well and requires decades of work. Building ongoing relationships and partnerships in community settings takes time and commitment, but it will build trust and help with sustainability.
3. **Pay attention to intervention exposure, and ensure that sufficient levels are achieved.** Strategies include monitoring intervention delivery, setting standards from the beginning, and modifying plans if the standards are not achieved (e.g., the number of stores to be included or the number of foods to be stocked to realize success).
4. **Work at multiple levels of the food system (i.e., consumers, retailers, suppliers, policy makers).** Different foods, such as healthy produce vs. a bag of chips, will have different distribution systems.
5. **Consider working at the policy level to support environmental interventions.** Doing so can help scale interventions beyond 10 or 20 stores. Digital strategies such as simulation models can also help in decision making and policy assessment by showing the expected benefits.

SOURCE: Presented by Joel Gittelsohn on August 16, 2023.

DISCUSSION

Speakers and participants focused on creating opportunities to bridge communication between retailers and the community and to improve access to alternative sources of produce, such as canned and frozen options. Gittelsohn said his group facilitates conversations as part of its community engagement process and identifies foods that are culturally acceptable for promotion in the stores. But a large part of this community engagement happens during the intervention itself, he stressed, such as by catching someone at the store when they are about to decide on purchases and using strategies such as taste testing. Laska added that it is not uncommon for store operators and customers to have different cultural or racial backgrounds, so it is important to ensure a common understanding of products. Gittelsohn agreed, sharing an example from his initial work in Baltimore in which around 70 percent of small store owners were Korean American, but their customers were primarily African American. There was a range of relationships, he noted, but many experienced challenges in communication.

With respect to produce, Gittelsohn asserted that fresh produce is highly overrated, pointing out that frozen produce is just as good with similar nutrient levels, but it can be much easier to provide to more remote locations. Essel noted that access to fresh produce is also an issue of equity, and many families want items they feel they cannot access. The Special Supplemental Nutrition Program for Women, Infants, and Children and Supplemental Nutrition Assistance Program (SNAP) give families expanded options, he observed, but he agreed that fresh items are overemphasized and too little emphasis is placed on the cost savings that can be realized by purchasing other options.

ROLES OF COMMUNITY-BASED ORGANIZATIONS

Beyond retailers and health care systems, community organizations around the country play important roles in improving access to healthy foods for families and individuals, especially those at lower income levels. Several speakers highlighted initiatives and potential opportunities from the work of food-focused community-based organizations.

Feeding Texas

Celia Cole, Feeding Texas, introduced the organization's work supporting 21 food banks across the state, noting that millions of Texans participate in food bank programs every year that are offered through a network of 3,000 community partners throughout Texas. While she acknowledged that it is not possible to "food bank our way out of hunger," Feeding Texas is leveraging its core strengths beyond meal provision to implement strategies that can improve overall health and well-being. Not only does the organization's network have a vast infrastructure of warehouses and cold storage facilities, but it also has a strong logistics capacity and maintains relationships across the food industry so it can move food where it needs to go at low or no cost. Approximately 4 million Texans participate in food bank programs every year, Cole explained, and each participant visits the food bank about seven times each year, which translates to 28 million opportunities to gain insight from the people being served. She shared three key strategies by which Feeding Texas is connecting food access with health.

The organization's first strategy involves ensuring that the food being distributed is as healthy as possible, with a focus on fresh produce. Cole explained that Texas grows an abundance of produce, and much of it goes to waste every year because of imperfections or market conditions. Food banks and Feeding Texas have agreements with growers across the state, she explained, to salvage surplus produce that cannot make it to market, providing a cost-effective way to increase access to produce in low-income communities. The difficulty many Texans face in accessing fresh produce is not just related to money, she observed, noting that many people live in a food desert or an area without access to healthy food. Feeding Texas also uses approaches such as mobile food delivery and home delivery for people who cannot get to a store and connects families to SNAP and other services that can increase their food resources. Feeding Texas has 120 trained case assistance navigators across the state at food banks to help people navigate the complex process of applying for SNAP and other benefits.

Cole described her organization's second strategy as providing nutrition education. Feeding Texas has a cadre of dieticians who can help people make healthier food choices. Approaches used to this end include, for example, education in food budgeting, cooking classes, and healthy choice pantries. The focus, Cole added, is always on interventions that combine healthy food choices with education to change behaviors, which Feeding Texas has found to be most effective.

Finally, Cole highlighted her organization's newer role in partnerships with health care providers, hospitals, and clinics to identify and treat food insecurity. This strategy ranges from identifying and diagnosing food insecurity to making referrals to food banks, assistance with benefit programs, and even writing food prescriptions for specific meals.

In terms of future direction, Cole said Feeding Texas is focusing on working with managed care organizations to develop scalable approaches to value-based care and reimbursement models that would create funding to sustain this role. In closing, she, emphasized the importance of public policy and systems interventions to address food insecurity and its root causes. She highlighted the opportunity offered by the upcoming farm bill to address the adequacy of SNAP benefits, as well as whom the program is serving and how people use the benefits. She argued that both strengthening other income support programs and creating good jobs are inextricably linked to direct food assistance and can indirectly affect food security for families, making these important areas on which to focus policy advocacy.

FoodCorps

Robert S. Harvey, FoodCorps, described the organization's recent focus on a theory of change that prioritizes efforts targeting the school system to influence connections between food and health. He explained that Food-Corps grounds itself in the belief that if young people are to be agents of their own bodies, interventions must focus on the place where they spend the most time. Specifically, FoodCorps targets the school cafeteria, the largest food infrastructure such efforts can impact, one that Harvey asserted is often overlooked as a potential target. He pointed out that there are seven times more school cafeterias in the United States than there are McDonald's restaurants. FoodCorps believes, Harvey elaborated, that it has an opportunity to radically transform the ways in which young people, especially people of color, can counter the impact of deep systemic racism through food. The organization seeks to transform "systemic and intergenerational food disease" through three approaches. Describing FoodCorps' first approach, Harvey noted that its direct services reach about half a million people daily. FoodCorps holds a national orientation to train service members and then deploys them to schools across 17 states and the District of Columbia, providing weekly food education lessons. The second strategy is policy work at the local, state, and federal levels, Harvey continued, encouraging states to offer nourishing meals for all students. A core aspect of this policy work is supporting local procurement, he added, and devising ways in which school districts can work alongside local farmers to build a cyclical ecosystem. This part of the organization's work serves more than 10 million young people. Finally, the organization's third approach involves digital advocacy and campaigns, focused on family engagement so as to include caregivers in the journey toward food justice and food literacy.

Wholesome Wave

Brent Ling, Wholesome Wave, echoed the observations of previous speakers regarding the highly complex food system, but argued that much is to be gained by focusing on the demand side of the system. He explained that Wholesome Wave was founded 16 years ago by a food business chef who knew the industry but was facing challenges related to diabetes within his own family. The organization's founders, he said, wanted to address the market failure of the lack of availability of healthy, high-quality produce. Since then, he continued, it has learned that shoppers do not want to be treated differently just because they have low income.

Ling went on to explain that Wholesome Wave's early work spurred the creation of the Gus Schumacher Nutrition Incentive Program (GusNIP), allowing SNAP benefits to be doubled for purchases at farmers' markets as a permanent feature of U.S. Department of Agriculture (USDA) policy. However, he noted, SNAP shoppers are often required to go to a special booth to get validated and receive tokens. Vendors then need to know which tokens are eligible for which food items, and when the tokens are used to pay, it is a public sign that these customers are living with low income. According to Ling, these barriers may impede easy access to a market. Ling concluded by asserting that everyone should be able to participate in the same food economy and be able to access healthy food in the same way.

DISCUSSION

Discussion centered on relationships with the health care system and linkages between food programs and health outcomes. In response to the opportunity challenges presented by the Centers for Medicare & Medicaid Services decree regarding screening for social determinants of health, Cole supported recognition of this link and argued that systems and providers need to start building partnerships and infrastructure to facilitate these types of referrals. She added that food banks need to secure resources and partnerships to meet the increasing demand for food, as well as provide the wraparound services needed to advance economic stability and mobility.

Regarding food program findings that relate to health outcomes, Harvey stated that FoodCorps is currently reevaluating its core metrics but has found that young people who have had 10 hours of FoodCorps direct instruction have three times the produce intake of those not having received that instruction. He also highlighted the organization's measurement of a sense of belonging, finding that young people feel as though they belong in their school environment more when they are familiar with the foods on the cafeteria menu.

Ling said that Wholesome Wave is preparing to release findings from its produce prescription program showing significant improvements in blood pressure, hemoglobin A1C (blood glucose), food security, and positive health care engagement and support for the program by patients. He also referenced the third-year impact findings from GusNIP showing that participants' fruit and vegetable consumption increased to a level above that of the average American. Thus the program not only bridged the existing income disparity in this regard but also surpassed it (Gretchen Swanson Center et al., 2023).

Cole added that measurement has been challenging for Feeding Texas, and the organization is working to better document outcomes in addition to outputs. Feeding Texas wants to know if it is truly moving the needle when it comes to food insecurity and advancing economic mobility for the people it serves.

Ling commented that it is an immense burden for a community-based organization to conduct research in addition to the programs it offers. He added that much of an organization's programming is done in a research vacuum, so any time it is possible to align researchers' needs with an organization's needs, the research is likely to be more replicable and more useful to the community.

A final question was asked regarding the messaging about fresh versus frozen produce and how to close the gap in perception of what is good for people's health and how the food cycle can be transformed to minimize waste. Cole replied that Feeding Texas is working with partners on education about so-called ugly fruits and vegetables and what is perfectly edible and nutritious despite its appearance. Harvey and Ling added that letting participants and patients drive the narrative can be powerful in communicating stories and successes.

LEGAL AND POLICY CHALLENGES FOR INTERVENTION

Jennifer L. Pomeranz, New York University, shared legal and policy opportunities relevant to the workshop discussions and offered several prominent themes. First, she noted the power of experimentation at the state and local levels, which she said is important because in some states, such as Mississippi, state legislatures have withdrawn the ability of local governments to act. Regulatory agencies have been active participants in many of these conversations, she added, but their resources and their authority to act are also limited. The current food environment is nudging people toward unhealthy food, she observed, a point made numerous times during the workshop, and she raised the question of how the healthy option can be made the default. She added that healthy food comes in many forms, but questioned whether consumers can identify healthy food beyond items such as kale? Finally, while she acknowledged that gaps remain in determining how to help all consumers, she highlighted the need to focus on disparities and how to increase people's access to healthy foods. She shared research and policies related to online food retail, in-store retail, and food labeling, along with regulatory challenges.

Online Food Retail

Pomeranz began by observing that online purchasing has increased in recent years, especially since the COVID-19 pandemic. She shared a study looking at online food labeling that analyzed 10 products across nine retailers involved in the SNAP online purchasing pilot. The researchers found that the four key elements of nutrition facts, ingredients, common food allergens, and percent juice (where applicable) were present and legible for only about 36 percent of products, whereas voluntary marketing claims, such as nutrient content claims, were available for more than 63 percent of products (Pomeranz et al., 2022). Even allergen information, which is a safety issue, was not widely available on products. She added that there were gaps not only across products but also across retailers with respect to what information was available. The same problem can be seen across food products in online retail, said Pomeranz. She believes USDA can drive change to enable better access to important information for consumers, as it regulates SNAP retail stores and can make this requirement apply online. She acknowledged, however, that an act of Congress may be required to make it to happen. Pomeranz added that the U.S. Food and Drug Administration (FDA) regulates labeling, which also includes shelf tags. However, she noted, there are arguments over whether online food retail qualifies as labeling, and there is no clear direction on how FDA would regulate in this space. She called for a broader conversation and more research to develop a clear framework for dealing with this issue.

In-Store Retail

Many in-store retailers operate at a very low profit margin, stated Pomeranz, so it is important that any structural changes taking place in stores do not result in the stores' increasing the price of food or going out of business. She argued that a policy at the state and local levels focused particularly on checkout aisles and endcap displays would nudge consumers toward healthier options. The goal would be to move healthier food to these locations that encourage purchasing, leaving the unhealthy items, such as candy, in their specifically designated aisles. The general idea is that the policy must be based on nutrition criteria, she clarified, not marketing. She suggested that this could be achieved in two ways—through conditional licensing or direct regulation. For conditional licensing, the government could require a license to operate as a food retailer and mandate that, as a condition for maintaining the license, healthy food must be sold in the checkout aisles and endcaps. The second way, Pomerantz continued, would be through direct mandates, as has been done in Berkeley, California. Both approaches are legally feasible and available as ways to effect change,

Pomeranz maintained. There are also some self-regulatory opportunities in this context; Pomeranz gave the example of Raley's supermarket chain, which created a family-friendly checkout aisle to support consumers. She also highlighted pharmacies, as people often forget they are now SNAP-approved food stores, which can also self-regulate, as CVS did when it made the decision to ban tobacco products from all its stores.

Food Labeling

Moving on to food labeling, Pomeranz again raised the question of whether consumers can easily identify healthy foods. Based on several studies, she said, consumers are confused about what is healthy, and reducing this confusion is key to success. As an example, she noted that 29–47 percent of participants in one study incorrectly identified the less healthy "whole-grain" product as the healthier one—even with access to the nutrition facts label (Wilde et al., 2020). Thus, she maintained, there appears to be a great deal of misunderstanding when it comes to whole versus refined grains, such that it can be difficult for consumers to differentiate between products that contain primarily refined grains with one whole grain and actual whole-grain products. She emphasized that across studies, consumers underestimate the healthfulness of healthier products, so that even when they are available, many people cannot identify them. She cited another study related to popular fruit drink beverages marketed for children, which found that most caretaker-respondents could not identify the drinks with non-nutritive sweeteners, and many thought sweetened flavored waters had no sugar and unsweetened juices did (Harris and Pomeranz, 2021). Therefore, she argued, food labels need to be updated with clear information to prevent such consumer confusion.

Lastly, Pomeranz focused on toddler formula-type drinks targeted to ages 1–3 years. She cited the consensus of professional medical associations recommending against the use of these products, noting that they are unnecessary and expensive, yet they look very similar to infant formula. While labels on such toddler drinks make several structure/function claims, Pomeranz observed, FDA says it does not have the authority to regulate structure/function claims for food. So not only are parents giving these drinks to their toddlers unnecessarily believing they are a healthy choice, but also caregivers may make the mistake of giving them to their infants because of the similarity in packaging and aisle placement. Emphasizing how powerful marketing and labeling can be across products, Pomeranz added that according to one study, more than 50 percent of infant caregivers incorrectly believed infant formula was nutritionally better than breastmilk (Romo-Palafox et al., 2020). In conclusion, she advocated for more opportunities for cross-pollination among retailers, manufacturers, researchers, and community members and suggested maintaining a focus on institutionalizing programs through Congress to ensure their sustainability across presidential administrations. She stressed that correcting consumer confusion about labels is one of the main priorities for enabling people to make the choices they want for themselves and their family.

References

Adams, K. M., W. S. Butsch, and M. Kohlmeier. 2015. The state of nutrition education at U.S. medical schools. *Journal of Biomedical Education* 2015(4):1-7.

Aysola, J., E. Tahirovic, A. B. Troxel, D. A. Asch, K. Gangemi, A. T. Hodlofski, J. Zhu, and K. Volpp. 2018. A randomized controlled trial of opt-in versus opt-out enrollment into a diabetes behavioral intervention. *American Journal of Health Promotion* 32(3):745-752.

Caspi, C. E., M. R. Winkler, K. M. Lenk, L. J. Harnack, D. J. Erickson, and M. N. Laska. 2020. Store and neighborhood differences in retailer compliance with a local staple foods ordinance. *BMC Public Health* 20:172.

Chaloupka, F. J., L. M. Powell, and K. E. Warner. 2019. The use of excise taxes to reduce tobacco, alcohol, and sugary beverage consumption. *Annual Review of Public Health* 40(1):187-201.

Chong, M. F.-F. 2022. Dietary trajectories through the life course: Opportunities and challenges. *British Journal of Nutrition* 128(1):154-159.

Diabetes Prevention Program Research Group. 2002. Reduction in the incidence of type 2 diabetes with lifestyle intervention or metformin. *New England Journal of Medicine* 346(6):393-403.

Dietary Guidelines Advisory Committee. 2020. *Scientific report of the 2020 Dietary Guidelines Advisory Committee: Advisory report to the Secretary of Agriculture and the Secretary of Health and Human Services.* Washington, DC: U.S. Department of Agriculture, Agricultural Research Service.

Dominguez-Salas, P., S. Moore, M. Baker, A. W. Bergen, S. E. Cox, R. A. Dyer, A. J. Fulford, Y. Guan, E. Laritsky, M. J. Silver, G. E. Swan, S. H. Zeisel, S. M. Innis, R. A. Waterland, A. M. Prentice, and B. J. Hennig. 2014. Maternal nutrition at conception modulates DNA methylation of human metastable epialleles. *Nature Communications* 5:3746.

Gangrade, N., J. Figueroa, and T. M. Leak. 2021. Socioeconomic disparities in foods/beverages and nutrients consumed by U.S. adolescents when snacking: National Health and Nutrition Examination Survey 2005–2018. *Nutrients* 13(8):2530.

Gretchen Swanson Center for Nutrition, Fair Food Network, and USDA (U.S. Department of Agriculture) National Institute of Food and Agriculture. 2023. *Gus Schumacher Nutrition Incentive Program (GusNIP): Impact findings Y3: September 1, 2021 to August 31, 2022.* Nutrition Incentive Program Training, Technical Assistance, Evaluation and Information.

Gunasekara, C. J., and R. A. Waterland. 2019. A new era for epigenetic epidemiology. *Epigenomics* 11(15):1647-1649.

Gunasekara, C. J., C. A. Scott, E. Laritsky, M. S. Baker, H. MacKay, J. D. Duryea, N. J. Kessler, G. Hellenthal, A. C. Wood, K. R. Hodges, M. Gandhi, A. B. Hair, M. J. Silver, S. E. Moore, A. M. Prentice, Y. Li, R. Chen, C. Coarfa, and R. A. Waterland. 2019. A genomic atlas of systemic interindividual epigenetic variation in humans. *Genome Biology* 20(1):105.

Gunasekara, C. J., H. MacKay, C. A. Scott, S. Li, E. Laritsky, M. S. Baker, S. L. Grimm, G. Jun, Y. Li, R. Chen, J. L. Wiemels, C. Coarfa, and R. A. Waterland. 2023. Systemic interindividual epigenetic variation in humans is associated with transposable elements and under strong genetic control. *Genome Biology* 24(1):2.

Gundersen, C., M. Strayer, A. Dewey, M. Hake, and E. Engelhard. 2023. *Map the meal gap 2023: An analysis of county and congressional district food insecurity and county food cost in the United States in 2021.* Chicago, IL: Feeding America. https://nutritionincentivehub.org/media/2uwlf3ch/gusnip-y3-impact-findings-report.pdf (accessed October 22, 2023).

Harris, J. L., and J. L. Pomeranz. 2021. Misperceptions about added sugar, non-nutritive sweeteners and juice in popular children's drinks: Experimental and cross-sectional study with U.S. parents of young children (1–5 years). *Pediatric Obesity* 16(10):e12791.

Herforth A., A. Venkat, Y. Bai, L. Costlow, C. Holleman, and W. A. Masters. 2022. Methods and options to monitor the cost and affordability of a healthy diet globally. Background paper for *The State of Food Security and Nutrition in the World 2022.* Rome, Italy: Food and Agriculture Organization of the United Nations.

Herrick, K. A., J. L. Lerman, T. E. Pannucci, M. Zimmer, M. M. Shams-White, K. M. Mathieu, E. E. Stoody, and J. Reedy. 2023. Continuity, considerations, and future directions for the Healthy Eating Index-Toddlers-2020. *Journal of the Academy of Nutrition and Dietetics* 123(9):1298-1306.

Kumanyika, S. K. 2019. A framework for increasing equity impact in obesity prevention. *American Journal of Public Health* 109(10):1350-1357.

Lampe, J. W., Y. Huang, M. L. Neuhouser, L. F. Tinker, X. Song, D.A. Schoeller, S. Kim, D. Raftery, C. Di, C. Zheng, Y. Schwarz, L. Van Horn, C. A. Thomson, Y. Mossavar-Rahmani, S. A. Beresford, and R. L. Prentice. 2017. Dietary biomarker evaluation in a controlled feeding study in women from the Women's Health Initiative cohort. *American Journal of Clinical Nutrition* 105(2):466-475.

Laska, M. N., C. E. Caspi, K. Lenk, S. G. Moe, J. E. Pelletier, L. J. Harnack, and D. J. Erickson. 2019. Evaluation of the first U.S. staple foods ordinance: Impact on nutritional quality of food store offerings, customer purchases and home food environments. *International Journal of Behavioral Nutrition and Physical Activity* 16(1):83.

Lerman, J. L., K. A. Herrick, T. E. Pannucci, M. M. Shams-White, L. L. Kahle, M. Zimmer, K. M. Mathieu, E. E. Stoody, and J. Reedy. 2023. Evaluation of the Healthy Eating Index-Toddlers-2020. *Journal of the Academy of Nutrition and Dietetics* 123(9):1307-1319.

Li, J., M. Guasch-Ferré, W. Chung, M. Ruiz-Canela, E. Toledo, D. Corella, S. N. Bhupathiraju, D. K. Tobias, F. K. Tabung, J. Hu, T. Zhao, C. Turman, Y. A. Feng, C. B. Clish, L. Mucci, A. H. Eliassen, K. H. Costenbader, E. W. Karlson, B. M. Wolpin, A. Ascherio, E. B. Rimm, J. E. Manson, L. Qi, M. Á. Martínez-González, J. Salas-Salvadó, F. B. Hu, and L. Liang. 2020. The Mediterranean diet, plasma metabolome, and cardiovascular disease risk. *European Heart Journal* 41(28):2645-2656.

Liese, A. D., S. M. Krebs-Smith, A. F. Subar, S. M. George, B. E. Harmon, M. L. Neuhouser, C. J. Boushey, T. E. Schap, and J. Reedy. 2015. The dietary patterns methods project: Synthesis of findings across cohorts and relevance to dietary guidance. *Journal of Nutrition* 145(3):393-402.

Liu, J., Y. Li, D. Zhang, S. S. Yi, and J. Liu. 2022. Trends in prediabetes among youths in the U.S. from 1999 through 2018. *JAMA Pediatrics* 176(6):608-611.

Maskarinec, G., M. A. J. Hullar, K. R. Monroe, J. A. Shepherd, J. Hunt, T. W. Randolph, L. R. Wilkens, C. J. Boushey, L. Le Marchand, U. Lim, and J. W. Lampe. 2019. Fecal microbial diversity and structure are associated with diet quality in the multiethnic cohort adiposity phenotype study. *Journal of Nutrition* 149(9):1575-1584.

McCullough, M. L., M. L. Maliniak, V. L. Stevens, B. D. Carter, R. A. Hodge, and Y. Wang. 2019. Metabolomic markers of healthy dietary patterns in U.S. postmenopausal women. *American Journal of Clinical Nutrition* 109(5):1439-1451.

Neuhouser, M. L., M. Pettinger, J. W. Lampe, L. F. Tinker, S. M. George, J. Reedy, X. Song, B. Thyagarajan, S. A. Beresford, and R. L. Prentice. 2021. Novel application of nutritional biomarkers from a controlled feeding study and an observational study to characterization of dietary patterns in postmenopausal women. *American Journal of Epidemiology* 190(11):2461-2473.

Olarte, D. A., J. Petimar, P. James, K. Cooksey-Stowers, S. B. Cash, E. B. Rimm, C. D. Economos, M. Rohmann, J. C. Blossom, Y. Chen, R. Deo, and J. F. W. Cohen. 2023. Trends in quick-service restaurants near public schools in the United States: Differences by community, school, and student characteristics. *Journal of the Academy of Nutrition and Dietetics* 123(6):923-932.

Palma, M. A., M. S. Segovia, B. Kassas, L. A. Ribera, and C. R. Hall. 2018. Self-control: Knowledge or perishable resource? *Journal of Economic Behavior & Organization* 145:80-94.

Pannucci, T. E., J. L. Lerman, K. A. Herrick, M. M. Shams-White, M. Zimmer, K. M. Mathieu, E. E. Stoody, and J. Reedy. 2023. Development of the Healthy Eating Index-Toddlers-2020. *Journal of the Academy of Nutrition and Dietetics* 123(9):1289-1297.

Peters, B. A., J. Xing, G. C. Chen, M. Usyk, Z. Wang, A. C. McClain, B. Thyagarajan, M. L. Daviglus, C. Sotres-Alvarez, F. B. Hu, R. Knight, R. D. Burk, R. C. Kaplan, and Q. Qi. 2023. Healthy dietary patterns are associated with the gut microbiome in the Hispanic Community Health Study/Study of Latinos. *American Journal of Clinical Nutrition* 117(3):540-552.

Plassmann, H., J. O'Doherty, B. Shiv, and A. Rangel. 2008. Marketing actions can modulate neural representations of experienced pleasantness. *Proceedings of the National Academy of Sciences* 105(3):1050-1054.

Pomeranz, J. L., S. B. Cash, M. Springer, I. M. Del Giudice, and D. Mozaffarian. 2022. Opportunities to address the failure of online food retailers to ensure access to required food labelling information in the USA. *Public Health Nutrition* 25(5):1-9.

Rebholz, C. M., A. H. Lichtenstein, Z. Zheng, L. J. Appel, and J. Coresh. 2018. Serum untargeted metabolomic profile of the Dietary Approaches to Stop Hypertension (DASH) dietary pattern. *American Journal of Clinical Nutrition* 108(2):243-255.

Roberto, C. A., H. G. Lawman, M. T. LeVasseur, N. Mitra, A. Peterhans, B. Herring, and S. N. Bleich. 2019. Association of a beverage tax on sugar-sweetened and artificially sweetened beverages with changes in beverage prices and sales at chain retailers in a large urban setting. *Journal of the American Medical Association* 321(18):1799-1810.

Romo-Palafox, M. J., J. L. Pomeranz, and J. L. Harris. 2020. Infant formula and toddler milk marketing and caregiver's provision to young children. *Maternal & Child Nutrition* 16(3):e12962.

Satia, J. A. 2009. Diet-related disparities: Understanding the problem and accelerating solutions. *Journal of the American Diet Association* 109(4):610-615.

Shams-White, M. M., T. E. Pannucci, J. L. Lerman, K. A. Herrick, M. Zimmer, K. Meyers Mathieu, E. E. Stoody, and J. Reedy. 2023. Healthy Eating Index-2020: Review and update process to reflect the dietary guidelines for Americans, 2020–2025. *Journal of the Academy of Nutrition and Dietetics* 123(9):1280-1288.

U.S. Bureau of Labor Statistics. *Consumer price index for all urban consumers: Food at home in U.S. city average [CUSR0000SAF11].* FRED (Federal Reserve Bank of St. Louis). https://fred.stlouisfed.org/series/CUSR0000SAF11 (accessed August 5, 2023).

Wang, P., M. Song, A. H. Eliassen, M. Wang, T. T. Fung, S. K. Clinton, E. B. Rimm, F. B. Hu, W. C. Willett, F. K. Tabung, and E. L. Giovannucci. 2023. Optimal dietary patterns for prevention of chronic disease. *Nature Medicine* 29(3):719-728.

Waterland, R. A., and C. Garza. 1999. Potential mechanisms of metabolic imprinting that lead to chronic disease. *American Journal of Clinical Nutrition* 69(2):179-197.

Waterland, R. A., and R. L. Jirtle. 2003. Transposable elements: Targets for early nutritional effects on epigenetic gene regulation. *Molecular and Cellular Biology* 23(15):5293-5300.

Waterland, R. A., R. Kellermayer, E. Laritsky, P. Rayco-Solon, R. A. Harris, M. Travisano, W. Zhang, M. S. Torskaya, J. Zhang, L. Shen, M. J. Manary, and A. M. Prentice. 2010. Season of conception in rural Gambia affects DNA methylation at putative human metastable epialleles. *pLoS Genetics* 6(12):e1001252.

Wilde, P., J. L. Pomeranz, L. J. Lizewski, and F. F. Zhang. 2020. Consumer confusion about wholegrain content and healthfulness in product labels: A discrete choice experiment and comprehension assessment. *Public Health Nutrition* 23(18):3324-3331.

Wolfson, J. A., and C. W. Leung. 2020. Food insecurity and COVID-19: Disparities in early effects for U.S. adults. *Nutrients* 12(6):1648.

Wolfson, J. A., C. W. Leung, and A. Moran. 2021. Meeting the moment: Policy changes to strengthen SNAP and improve health. *Milbank Quarterly Opinion.*

Wolfson, J. A., H. Posluszny, S. Kronsteiner-Gicevic, W. Willett, and C. W. Leung. 2022. Food insecurity and less frequent cooking dinner at home are associated with lower diet quality in a national sample of low-income adults in the United States during the initial months of the Coronavirus Disease 2019 pandemic. *Journal of the Academy of Nutrition and Dietetics* 122(10):1893-1902.

Wolgast, H., M. M. Halverson, N. Kennedy, I. Gallard, and A. Karpyn. 2022. Encouraging healthier food and beverage purchasing and consumption: A review of interventions within grocery retail settings. *International Journal of Environmental Research and Public Health* 19(23):e16107.

Zhu, Y., N. Jain, J. Normington, N. Holschuh, and L. M. Sanders. 2022. Ready-to-eat cereal is an affordable breakfast option associated with better nutrient intake and diet quality in the U.S. population. *Frontiers Nutrition* 9:e1088080.

Appendix A

Workshop Agenda

Dietary Patterns to Prevent and Manage Diet-Related Disease
Across the Lifespan

August 15–16, 2023

August 15, 2023

10:00 AM   Opening Remarks and Overview of Workshop Focus
            Robin A. McKinnon, U.S. Food and Drug Administration;
            Planning Committee Chair

            SESSION 1—SETTING THE STAGE ON DIETARY
            PATTERNS AND CHRONIC DISEASE

10:15 AM   Dietary Pattern Assessment Across the Life Course
            Jill Reedy, National Institutes of Health

10:40 AM   Beyond Traditional Nutrition Markers for Assessing
            Dietary Quality and Chronic Disease Risk
            Johanna Lampe, Fred Hutchinson Cancer Center

11:05 AM   Review of the Evidence on Dietary Patterns and Chronic
            Disease Across the Lifespan
            Edward L. Giovannucci, Harvard University

11:30 AM   Break

11:40 AM   Developmental Origins of Chronic Disease and the
           Influence of Diet
           Robert Waterland, U.S. Department of Agriculture
           Agricultural Research Service Children's Nutrition
           Research Center, Baylor College of Medicine

12:05 PM   Q&A and Discussion

12:30 PM   Lunch Break

SESSION 2—DIMENSIONS OF FOOD CHOICE AND INFLUENCES ON DIETARY PATTERNS

1:00 PM   Understanding and Intervening on Inequities in Nutrition
           and Health
           Cindy Leung, Harvard University
           Tashara M. Leak, Cornell University

1:40 PM   Q&A and Discussion

1:55 PM   Food Choice and Access to Healthy Diets: Evidence from
           Food Prices and Diet Costs Worldwide
           William Masters, Tufts University

2:15 PM   Improving Dietary Health Through Behavioral Economics
           Kevin Volpp, University of Pennsylvania

2:35 PM   Q&A and Discussion

2:50 PM   The Role of Industry and Consumer Perspectives
           Marco A. Palma, Texas A&M University
           Beatrice Abiero, Instacart
           Sarah Ludmer, Kellogg Company
           Josh Hix, Season Health

3:30 PM   Adjourn Day 1

August 16, 2023

10:00 AM   Welcome and Workshop Recap
            Robin A. McKinnon, U.S. Food and Drug Administration;
            Planning Committee Chair

SESSION 3—TRANSLATING SOLUTIONS FOR THE FUTURE
OF DIETARY PATTERNS AND CHRONIC DISEASE

10:10 AM   Lessons Learned from Research to Improve the
            Healthfulness of Food Environments
            Melissa Laska, University of Minnesota

10:30 AM   Lessons Learned from Research to Improve Food
            Environments for Infants and Children in DC
            Kofi D. Essel, Elevance Health

10:50 AM   Lessons Learned from Research to Improve Food
            Environments for Adults in Baltimore
            Joel Gittelsohn, Johns Hopkins University

11:10 AM   Q&A and Discussion

11:20 AM   Community-Based Organization Experiences
            Celia Cole, Feeding Texas
            Robert S. Harvey, FoodCorps
            Brent Ling, Wholesome Wave

12:00 PM   Legal and Policy Challenges for Intervention
            Jennifer L. Pomeranz, New York University

12:20 PM   Q&A and Discussion

12:30 PM   Adjourn Workshop

Appendix B

Acronyms and Abbreviations

AHA	American Hospital Association
CoRSIV	correlated regions of systemic interindividual epigenetic variation
DASH	Dietary Approaches to Stop Hypertension
DGA	*Dietary Guidelines for Americans*
DoHAD	developmental origins of health and disease
FDA	U.S. Food and Drug Administration
FLiP	Family Lifestyle Program
GusNIP	Gus Schumacher Nutrition Incentive Program
HDB	Healthy Diet Basket
HEI	Healthy Eating Index
SES	socioeconomic status
SNAP	Supplemental Nutrition Assistance Program
USDA	U.S. Department of Agriculture
WIC	Special Supplemental Nutrition Program for Women, Infants, and Children

Appendix C

Biographical Sketches of Workshop Speakers and Planning Committee Members

Beatrice Abiero, Ph.D., is a policy research leader at Instacart, a leading grocery technology company in North America. She is passionate about researching health and food access and prides herself on being a creative and results-oriented thought leader. Dr. Abiero manages external research partnerships, directs large-scale research studies, and engages in coalition building for Instacart's Policy and Government Affairs team. She leverages her extensive experience in social science research to provide actionable insights that inform Instacart's policy and business development, ballot initiatives, and strategic priorities. Prior to joining Instacart, Dr. Abiero led large-scale analyses and reports as key analytics manager for a $31.8 million patient experience and satisfaction survey program to inform Military Health System stakeholders on how to improve care for 4.5 million beneficiaries. Her research resulted in peer-reviewed publications and numerous high-profile reports that provided military surgeon generals and C-suite health executives with strategies for enhancing quality care and patient experience. Dr. Abiero earned a dual-title Ph.D. in health policy and administration and demography from The Pennsylvania State University.

Alison Brown, Ph.D., M.S., R.D.N., serves as a program director at the National Heart, Lung, and Blood Institute, National Institutes of Health, where her work centers on the social determinants of health and nutrition health disparities. She is a public health nutrition researcher committed to addressing diet-related health disparities through research, community engagement and empowerment, and systems change. Dr. Brown's past research explored immigrant health and diet and cardiovascular disease outcomes. She also served as past chair of the National Organization of Blacks in Dietetics and Nutrition and as adjunct faculty at Prince George's Community College. She is a former science and technology policy fellow of the American Association for the Advancement of Science, Academy of Nutrition and Dietetics diversity leader, American Society of Nutrition science policy fellow, and board chair of a community-owned grocery store in Boston. In 2018, she was honored as a 40 under 40 Leader in Minority Health by the National Minority Quality Forum. Dr. Brown received a bachelor of science in chemistry from Spelman College and thereafter completed her master of science from Columbia University in nutrition and applied physiology. She then earned her Ph.D. from Tufts University's Friedman School of Nutrition Science and Policy.

Celia Cole, M.A., is chief executive officer of Feeding Texas, the state association of food banks. The Feeding Texas network works collaboratively with more than 3,000 local partners to increase access to nutritious food for people facing hunger, improve community nutrition, mitigate the root causes of hunger, and strengthen crisis response. Prior to Feeding Texas, Ms. Cole served as senior food policy analyst at Every Texas, a public policy research and advocacy organization. Over the course of her 25-year career, she has led advocacy campaigns to strengthen federal nutrition programs, established a statewide produce collaborative to increase access to fresh produce, and forged cross-sector partnerships with diverse stakeholders to increase food security, improve health outcomes, and build a robust response to hunger. Over the last 2 years, she has coordinated the network's response to the COVID-19 pandemic, marshaling new resources to food banks that have enabled them to double their food distribution to meet the surge in demand from communities devastated by the economic and health crisis. Ms. Cole holds a bachelor's degree in art history from Columbia University and a master's degree from the Institute of Latin American Studies at The University of Texas at Austin.

Cindy Davis, Ph.D., serves as national program leader for the program in human nutrition conducted by the U.S. Department of Agriculture (USDA) Agricultural Research Service. In this role, she helps direct the scientific program for six Human Nutrition Research Centers. Prior to joining USDA, she was director of grants and extramural activities in the Office of Dietary Supplements (ODS), where she actively engaged and encouraged partnerships with other National Institutes of Health (NIH) Institutes and Centers to develop a portfolio that advances both nutritional and botanical dietary supplement research for optimizing public health. Dr. Davis is also actively involved in a number of government working groups focused on the microbiome, including being a cofounder and cochair of the Joint

Agency Microbiome working group (NIH, U.S. Food and Drug Administration, National Institute of Standards and Technology, and USDA). Before moving to ODS, she was a program director in the Nutritional Sciences Research Group at the National Cancer Institute. Dr. Davis completed her postdoctoral training at the Laboratory of Experimental Carcinogenesis at the National Cancer Institute. She then joined the Grand Forks Human Nutrition Research Center, USDA, as a research nutritionist. In 2000, Dr. Davis received a Presidential Early Career Award for Scientists and Engineers and was named the USDA Early Career Scientist. She is a supplement editor for the *Journal of Nutrition*, assistant editor for *Nutrition Reviews*, and a member of the editorial board for *Advances in Nutrition*. Dr. Davis received her Ph.D. in nutrition with a minor in human cancer biology from the University of Wisconsin–Madison.

Kofi D. Essel, M.D., M.P.H., FAAP, is inaugural food-as-medicine program director at Elevance Health. As a core member of the Health Outcomes Organization team, he works to coordinate with the broader social impact strategy, health equity, and medical policy initiatives throughout the enterprise. He leads efforts in designing innovative approaches to address diet-related chronic diseases and social risk using novel food interventions. Dr. Essel is a board-certified community pediatrician at Children's National Hospital in Washington, DC. He has dedicated his career to advocacy/research around health care and public health workforce training, health disparities, and community engagement, with expertise and national recognition in the areas of addressing diet-related chronic disease and food insecurity with patients and families. Dr. Essel sits on the board of directors for the Food Research and Action Center (FRAC), serves as a physician advisor for the Partnership for a Healthier America's "Veggies Early & Often" campaign, and is a member of the executive committee for the American Academy of Pediatrics (AAP) Section on Obesity. He also coauthored a national toolkit for pediatric providers on addressing food insecurity in their clinical settings with the AAP and FRAC. Dr. Essel earned his M.D. and M.P.H. in epidemiology from The George Washington University.

Mario Ferruzzi, Ph.D., M.S., is professor and chief of the section of Developmental Nutrition in the Department of Pediatrics at the University of Arkansas for Medical Sciences. He also serves as director of the Arkansas Children's Nutrition Center, a partnership between the Arkansas Children's Research Institute and the U.S. Department of Agriculture/Agricultural Research Service. Dr. Ferruzzi joined the Arkansas Children's Nutrition Center as director in 2021, having previously served as David H. Murdock distinguished professor at North Carolina State University's Plants for Human Health Institute (2016–2021) and as professor of food science and nutrition science at Purdue University (2004–2016). His research interests are at the interface of agriculture, food, and nutrition sciences in the study of food matrix and processing factors that influence micronutrient and phytochemical bioavailability, metabolism, and impact to human health. He has a particular interest in strategies that can be leveraged to improve the nutritional and functional quality of food products for at-risk populations. Dr. Ferruzzi earned his M.S. and Ph.D. in food science and nutrition from The Ohio State University.

Edward L. Giovannucci, M.D., Sc.D., is professor of nutrition and epidemiology at Harvard T. H. Chan School of Public Health. Over the past three decades, his work has been based largely on prospective cohort studies, such as the Nurses' Health Study I & II and the Health Professionals Follow-Up Study. His research focuses on how nutritional, lifestyle and genetic factors affect the risk of development and progression of various malignancies, especially those of the large intestine, other gastrointestinal cancers, and prostate cancer. A specific interest has been understanding etiologic mechanisms underlying the relation between diet, physical activity, body weight and composition, and metabolic dysfunction and cancer risk. Dr. Giovannucci currently serves as an American Cancer Society clinical researcher professor. Fourteen of his former primary pre- or postdoctoral mentees are full professors and 11 are assistant/associate professors. Dr. Giovannucci graduated from Harvard University in 1980, and he received his M.D. from the University of Pittsburgh in 1984. He did his residency in anatomic pathology at the University of Connecticut and completed his Sc.D. in epidemiology from the Harvard T. H. Chan School of Public Health in 1992.

Joel Gittelsohn, Ph.D., M.S., is professor in the Department of International Health at the Johns Hopkins Bloomberg School of Public Health. He is a public health nutritionist and medical anthropologist, who focuses on the primary prevention of chronic disease in disadvantaged communities. With more than 300 publications, Dr. Gittelsohn has led multiple intervention trials aimed at improving the food environment and providing education needed to support healthy food choices and reduce obesity and diabetes in Native communities, Baltimore City, and Pacific Islander communities. He has conducted a series of intervention trials with corner stores, carryouts, wholesalers, churches, and recreation centers in Baltimore City. Recently, he has begun to use systems science methods in his work to simulate the impact and unexpected consequences of policies to improve the urban food environment, and he is developing an app to improve the distribution of healthy foods to food sources located in low-income neighborhoods of Baltimore. Dr. Gittelsohn currently leads grants for improving the food environment by working with independently owned restaurants, retail food stores, and food pantries. He earned his Ph.D. in medical anthropology from the University of Connecticut.

Robert S. Harvey, D.Min., M.T.S., is president of FoodCorps and an educator and community leader pursuing a vision of justice, equity, and love. FoodCorps is a national organization committed to ensuring that all the nation's children have access to nourishing food in schools at the intersection of community-building and racial and economic justice. He also holds a visiting professorship in the practice of public leadership. Prior to FoodCorps, Dr. Harvey served as superintendent of East Harlem Scholars Academies, a community-based network of public charter schools, and as chief academic officer of East Harlem Tutorial Program (EHTP) in New York City. Before that, he served as chief operating officer, head of school, dean of students, and classroom teacher at EHTP. Dr. Harvey is author of *Abolitionist Leadership in Schools: Undoing Systemic Injustice through Communally Consciousness Education* (Routledge, 2021), which explores school leadership and racial equity through the moral arc of an abolitionist lineage, and *Teaching as Protest: Emancipating Classrooms through Racial Consciousness* (Routledge, 2022), which frames philosophical and practical pedagogy that centers freeing teaching and learning spaces for students and teachers. He is a Pahara Institute Fellow, serves as chair of The Current Project Board of Directors, and is a member of the National Black Theatre Board of Directors. Dr. Harvey earned a master of theological studies from Harvard University and a doctor of ministry from the Memphis Theological Seminary.

Josh Hix, M.B.A., is cofounder and CEO of Season Health, the only integrated food-as-medicine platform that enables people to eat well and live well. By combining evidence-based clinical care with access to affordable medically tailored meals and groceries, Season Health empowers individuals and their families to make informed, sustainable choices, measurably improving both health outcomes and quality of life. Mr. Hix is also cofounder and former CEO of Plated, which shipped millions of meals to over 95 percent of the United States before being acquired by Albertsons grocery brands in 2017. He has a lifelong interest in health and nutrition. Mr. Hix received his B.S. in electrical engineering from the Georgia Institute of Technology and M.B.A. from Harvard Business School.

Johanna Lampe, Ph.D., R.D., is professor and associate division director in the Public Health Sciences Division at Fred Hutchinson Cancer Center and a research professor in the Nutritional Sciences Program and Department of Epidemiology at the University of Washington in Seattle. Her research focuses on the effect of diet on cancer susceptibility in humans and the effects of human genetic and gut microbiome variation in response to dietary constituents and dietary patterns. As part of several transdisciplinary collaborative studies, she also applies a variety of -omics approaches to the development of biomarkers of dietary exposure. Dr. Lampe has received several awards for her work, including the American Society for Nutrition Mary Swartz Rose Senior Investigator Award for research on the safety and efficacy of bioactive compounds for human health and the National Cancer Institute's Division of Cancer Prevention Stars in Nutrition and Cancer award, which recognizes research contributions in the field of nutrition and cancer. She earned her Ph.D. in nutrition from the University of Minnesota.

Melissa Laska, Ph.D., R.D., serves as McKnight distinguished professor at the University of Minnesota School of Public Health. Her expertise is in nutrition promotion, healthy food access, and nutrition inequities, and she has a broad background in community-informed prevention, intervention, and policy research. Over the past two decades, Dr. Laska has led a multifaceted research portfolio with the goal of realizing our potential to support healthy communities—particularly communities that have been historically under resourced—as well as individuals' autonomy in making healthy choices, including healthy food choices. Her interdisciplinary work has been supported by the National Institutes of Health, Centers for Disease Control and Prevention, and U.S. Department of Agriculture, and she has coauthored nearly 200 peer-reviewed publications to date. Dr. Laska is clinically trained as a registered dietitian. She completed her dietetic internship at Vanderbilt University and earned her Ph.D. from The University of North Carolina at Chapel Hill.

Tashara M. Leak, Ph.D., R.D., is associate professor in the Division of Nutritional Sciences and associate dean in the College of Human Ecology at Cornell University. She has a secondary appointment as associate professor of nutrition research in the Division of General Internal Medicine at Weill Cornell Medicine. Dr. Leak also serves as codirector of the Cornell Action Research Collaborative, which provides infrastructure for researchers, policy makers, and community partners to collaborate on pressing societal issues (e.g., food insecurity) across New York State. Regarding her research, Dr. Leak examines disparities in nutrition and health outcomes among U.S. adolescents and designs culturally inclusive interventions in New York City to address these inequities. Her research is predominately funded by grants from the U.S. Department of Agriculture and the National Institute on Minority Health and Health Disparities. Dr. Leak holds a Ph.D. in nutrition from the University of Minnesota Twin Cities and completed her postdoctoral training at the University of California, Berkeley School of Public Health.

Cindy Leung, Sc.D., M.P.H., is assistant professor of public health nutrition at the Harvard T. H. Chan School of Public Health. She is a nutrition epidemiologist with additional training in health psychology and health disparities research. Her program of research focuses on understanding structural determinants of diet-related health disparities in the United States with a particular focus on populations at risk of food insecurity. Her research has extensively examined the effects of food insecurity on dietary quality, health behaviors, and physical and mental health on populations across the life course using both quantitative and qualitative methods. Dr. Leung holds an M.P.H. from the University of California, Berkeley, and a Sc.D. in nutrition and epidemiology from Harvard University.

Brent Ling, M.S.P.H., serves as director of external affairs at Wholesome Wave. He is an advocate for health in all policy and a strong supporter of open and accessible government structures—this belief is rooted in over a decade of experience as a social-benefit small business owner, manager, investor, and frontline worker. Mr. Ling has been published in leading academic journals on topics of health and policy maker engagement. A longtime resident of the District of Columbia, he is a graduate of the schools of public health at Johns Hopkins University and Indiana University.

Sarah Ludmer, R.D., is senior director of well-being and regulatory for Kellogg Company. She has been appointed to the future leadership team of W. K. Kellogg Co. to serve as chief well-being and sustainable business officer when the company spins off in January 2024. Ms. Ludmer joined Kellogg Company in February 2014. Prior to becoming senior director in June 2019, she held several roles in nutrition and regulatory affairs, combining her passion for public health and love of consumers to unlock growth. In this capacity, she ensured strategic outcomes and helped brands positively impact both people and the planet while meeting the needs of their diverse range of consumers. Before joining Kellogg, Ms. Ludmer spent 5 years with Del Monte Foods in the research and quality team supporting both nutrition and regulatory affairs for pet and consumer goods. Prior to that, she spent 10 years in clinical practice building a strong foundation in nutrition and public health. She is a member of the Academy of Nutrition and Dietetics. Ms. Ling holds a B.S. in nutrition from The Pennsylvania State University, completed her dietetic internship at the Cleveland Clinic Foundation, and is a registered dietitian.

William Masters, Ph.D., M.A., is professor of food economics and policy in the Friedman School of Nutrition at Tufts University, where he leads the Food Prices for Nutrition project, which computes the cost and affordability of healthy diets, as well as the Innovative Metrics and Methods for

Agriculture and Nutrition Actions Fellowships program, among other initiatives. From 2011 to 2014, Dr. Masters served as chair of the Friedman School's Department of Food and Nutrition Policy, and before coming to Tufts was a faculty member in agricultural economics at Purdue University (1991–2010). He was also a lecturer or faculty member at the University of Zimbabwe (1989–1990), Harvard's Kennedy School of Government (2000), and Columbia University (2003–2004). Dr. Masters is coauthor of an undergraduate textbook, *Economics of Agricultural Development: World Food Systems and Resource Use* (Routledge, 4th ed., 2021) and former editor-in-chief of the journal *Agricultural Economics* (2006–2011). He was named an international fellow of the African Association of Agricultural Economists (2010) and elected fellow of the Agricultural and Applied Economics Association in 2020, from which he received the Bruce Gardner Memorial Prize for Applied Policy Analysis (2013), the Publication of Enduring Quality Award (2014), the Quality of Research Discovery Award (2019), and the Quality of Communications Award (2022). At Tufts, his courses on economics of agriculture, food, and nutrition were recognized with student-nominated, university-wide teaching awards in each of the past 2 years offered (2019 and 2022). Dr. Masters holds an M.A. and Ph.D. from the Food Research Institute at Stanford University.

Robin A. McKinnon, Ph.D., M.P.A., is senior advisor for nutrition policy at the U.S. Food and Drug Administration (FDA) Center for Food Safety and Applied Nutrition (CFSAN). She works to advance nutrition-related activities across CFSAN, including the FDA elements in the White House National Strategy on Hunger, Nutrition, and Health. Prior to joining the FDA, Dr. McKinnon was a health policy specialist at the National Cancer Institute, National Institutes of Health. She previously served on the planning committee for the 2009 workshop of the National Academies of Sciences, Engineering, and Medicine titled The Public Health Effects of Food Deserts; in 2021, she served on the planning committee for the National Academies workshop Challenges and Opportunities for Precision and Personalized Nutrition. Dr. McKinnon earned a master's degree in public administration from Harvard University in 2002 and a Ph.D. in public policy and administration from The George Washington University in 2009.

Emily Oken, M.D., M.P.H., is Alice Hamilton Professor and vice chair in the Department of Population Medicine at Harvard Medical School and the Harvard Pilgrim Health Care Institute and professor in the Department of Nutrition at the Harvard T. H. Chan School of Public Health. She directs the Division of Chronic Disease Research Across the Lifecourse within the Department of Population Medicine. Her research focuses on the influence of nutrition and other modifiable factors during pregnancy and early childhood on long-term maternal and child health, especially cardiometabolic health and cognitive development. Dr. Oken was a planning committee member for the 2020 workshop of the National Academies of Sciences, Engineering, and Medicine titled Nutrition During Pregnancy and Lactation: Exploring New Evidence. She served on the Technical Expert Collaborative 1 for the Dietary Guidance Development Project for Birth to 24 Months and Pregnancy and coauthored the work that came out of the committee. Dr. Oken obtained her master's degree in public health from the Harvard School of Public Health. She received her medical degree from Harvard Medical School in 1996, completed her internship and residency in internal medicine and pediatrics at the Harvard Combined Program, and completed her fellowship in general internal medicine at Harvard Medical School.

Marco A. Palma, Ph.D., M.S., is professor in the Department of Agricultural Economics at Texas A&M University. His areas of interest are consumer economics, experimental and behavioral economics, and neuroeconomics. Dr. Palma is a Texas A&M Presidential Impact Fellow and director of the Human Behavior Laboratory (HBL), a transdisciplinary facility that integrates state-of-the-art technology to measure neurophysiological responses of human decision making. The HBL aims to facilitate the integration of neurophysiological responses to traditional methods of studying human behavior to better understand, predict, and change behavior that improves people's health and well-being. Dr. Palma earned his M.S. in food and resource economics and Ph.D. from the University of Florida.

Jennifer L. Pomeranz, J.D., M.P.H., is associate professor in the Department of Public Health Policy and Management in the School of Global Public Health at New York University. She was previously director of legal initiatives at the Rudd Center for Food Policy and Obesity at Yale University (now the University of Connecticut Rudd Center for Food Policy & Health). Her research focuses on legal opportunities and barriers to enacting public health policies at the federal, state, and local levels with a primary focus on food and nutrition policy. Ms. Pomeranz is author of the book *Food Law for Public Health* and the first author of the book *Public Health Law in Practice*, published by Oxford University Press in 2016 and 2023, respectively. She has also authored dozens of peer-reviewed journal articles on policy and legal options for addressing products that cause harm, diet-related disease, and social injustices that lead to health disparities. Ms. Pomeranz earned her M.P.H. from the Harvard T. H. Chan School of Public Health and J.D. from Cornell Law School.

Jill Reedy, Ph.D., M.P.H., R.D., is chief of the Risk Factor Assessment Branch (RFAB) of the Epidemiology and Genomics Research Program

(EGRP) in the Division of Cancer Control and Population Sciences at the National Cancer Institute (NCI), National Institutes of Health (NIH). As branch chief, she oversees EGRP's research portfolio and initiatives that focus on dietary and physical activity assessment; methods, tools, technologies, and resources for risk factor assessment; and obesity policy research. Her scientific interests include different methodological approaches in dietary pattern analysis, dietary surveillance, obesity policy, new technologies for dietary assessment, and measures of the food environment. Dr. Reedy leads the Dietary Patterns Methods Project, a collaboration with investigators from three large U.S. cohorts, which aims to systematically examine index-based scoring systems using standardized methods with mortality outcomes. She partners with colleagues at the NCI, the U.S. Department of Agriculture, and the National Collaborative on Childhood Obesity Research to develop resources for researchers, including the Measures Registry, User Guides, Catalogue of Surveillance Systems, and the Healthy Eating Index. Dr. Reedy is a member of the Data Analysis Team for the 2020–2025 Dietary Guidelines Advisory Committee, and she has served in a similar capacity for past Dietary Guidelines. She serves on the Senior Leadership Group for the NIH Nutrition Research Task Force and leads several trans-NIH working groups, as well as the NIH Obesity Policy Research Grantees Network. Dr. Reedy earned a B.A. in foods and nutrition at Goshen College, an M.P.H. at the University of California, Berkeley, and a Ph.D. in nutrition at The University of North Carolina at Chapel Hill.

Rebecca Seguin-Fowler, Ph.D., M.S., R.D.N., L.D., CSCS, is associate director for the Texas A&M Institute for Advancing Health through Agriculture, where she leads the Healthy Living social and behavioral research program. She is also chief scientific officer for the Healthy Texas Institute, professor with tenure in the Department of Nutrition in the College of Agriculture & Life Sciences, and graduate faculty in the Department of Health Promotion and Community Health Sciences at the School of Public Health at Texas A&M University. Dr. Seguin-Fowler is also owner of StrongPeople, LLC, an organization that provides consulting services in the areas of nutrition, food, exercise, and wellness, as well as resources, such as trainings and curricula, to advance community health. She is recognized internationally for her expertise in behavioral intervention development for rural residents, low-income families, and older adults; food systems and food access interventions; civic engagement to catalyze policy, systems, and environmental change; and dissemination and implementation science. Dr. Seguin-Fowler has received numerous awards, including the Mead Johnson Award from the American Society for Nutrition; an Excellence Award from the Society of Behavioral Medicine; and most recently, the Friedman School Alumni Excellence in Nutrition Award from Tufts University. A registered and licensed dietitian, she received her bachelor's degree in clinical exercise physiology from Boston University and a master's degree in nutrition communication and doctorate in food policy and applied nutrition from Tufts University.

Jessica Smith, Ph.D., is senior principal scientist at Mars Wrigley, where she leads nutrition scientific and regulatory affairs for the North American region. Prior to joining Mars Wrigley in February 2022, she held various roles from 2015 to 2022 at General Mills' Bell Institute of Health and Nutrition. Before transitioning to the food industry, Dr. Smith began her career in academia by completing two postdoctoral fellowships at Laval University (Quebec, QC) and the Harvard T. H. Chan School of Public Health, where her research focused on the associations between diet, obesity, and chronic disease risk. She has a B.S. in nutrition from the University of Western Ontario (London, ON); an M.S. in nutrition from McGill University (Montreal, QC); and a Ph.D. in physiology from Laval University (Quebec, QC), where her thesis focused on the physiology of adipose tissue in obesity.

Kevin Volpp, M.D., Ph.D., is Mark V. Pauly Presidential Distinguished Professor of Medicine, Medical Ethics and Policy, and of health care management at the Perelman School of Medicine and the Wharton School at the University of Pennsylvania. He is also founding director of the Penn Center for Health Incentives and Behavioral Economics. His research focuses on the impact of financial and organizational incentives on health behavior and health outcomes. Dr. Volpp has been recognized by numerous awards, including the Alice S. Hersh Award from AcademyHealth, the *British Medical Journal* Group Award for Translating Research into Practice, outstanding paper of the year from multiple societies, the Presidential Early Career Award for Scientists and Engineers, and numerous others. He cocreated the Penn Way to Health platform, used to facilitate behavioral interventions, which has now been deployed in more than 200 studies by investigators from more than 20 universities, with participants in all 50 states. Dr. Volpp earned his bachelor's degree magna cum laude in biology from Harvard University and was a Rotary Scholar at Freie Universitat in Berlin, Germany, where he studied the organization of health care delivery in the former East Germany. He earned an M.D. from Perelman School of Medicine and a Ph.D. from the Wharton School, both at the University of Pennsylvania.

Robert Waterland, Ph.D., is professor at Baylor College of Medicine and is based in the U.S. Department of Agriculture/Agriculture Research Service Children's Nutrition Research Center in Houston, Texas. He holds faculty appointments in the Department of Pediatrics/Nutrition and the Department of Molecular & Human Genetics. Dr. Waterland's research focuses on understanding how nutrition during critical periods of prenatal and early postnatal development affects gene expression, metabolism, and chronic disease susceptibility in adulthood. His laboratory studies both mouse models and humans to elucidate the mechanisms by which early nutrition and other environmental influences affect the establishment and maintenance of epigenetic gene regulation, with a focus on DNA methylation. He serves on the council of the International Society for Developmental Origins of Health and Disease and various journal editorial boards. Dr. Waterland received his B.S. in physics from Virginia Polytechnic Institute and State University and worked for several years at the University of Pennsylvania, first with Britton Chance (biochemistry/biophysics), then with Albert Stunkard (clinical obesity research). After earning his Ph.D. in human nutrition from Cornell University (with Cutberto Garza), he conducted postdoctoral research in developmental genetics with Randy Jirtle at Duke University.

Fang Fang Zhang, Ph.D., M.D., is Neely Family Professor and associate professor at the Friedman School of Nutrition Science and Policy, Tufts University. She is a nutritional epidemiologist with expertise in assessing dietary intake patterns, trends, and disparities in the population, and conducting observational studies and clinical trials to investigate the role of nutrition in chronic disease prevention and control. Dr. Zhang's research interests also include quantifying preventable cancer burden associated with suboptimal diet and assessing the cost-effectiveness of population strategies for improving diet and reducing cancer burden and disparities in the United States, as well as evaluating strategies for integrating food and nutrition into health care. She is coleading the LASTING project, which is focused on assessing the impact of diet on four pillars (health, environment, cost, and society). Dr. Zhang is a recipient of the Eileen O'Neil Citation for Excellence in Teaching and an inaugural recipient of the Miriam E. Nelson Tisch Faculty Fellow from Tufts University. She received her M.D. from Fudan University Shanghai Medical College and her Ph.D. from Columbia University.

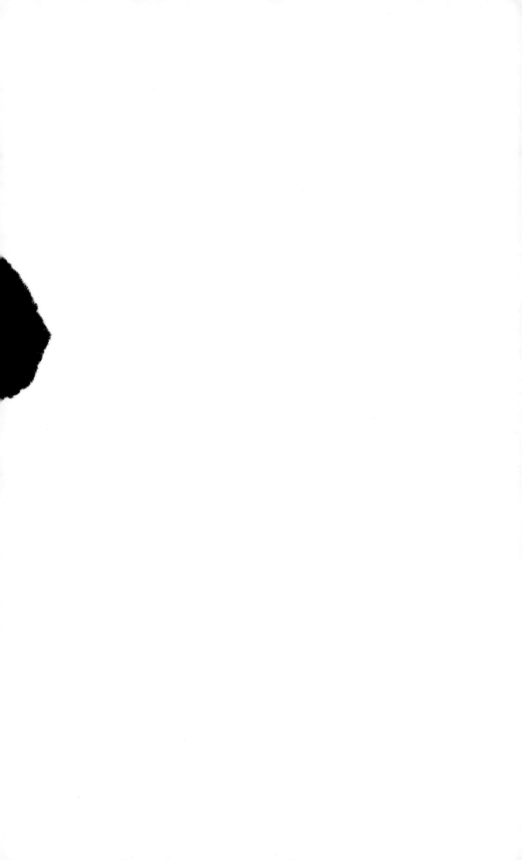